Don't Unplug

Don't Unplug

HOW TECHNOLOGY
SAVED MY LIFE
AND CAN SAVE
YOURS TOO

Chris Dancy

St. Martin's Press
New York

www.stmartins.com

Designed by Meryl Sussman Levavi

The Library of Congress Cataloging-in-Publication Data
is available upon request.

ISBN 978-1-250-15417-0 (hardcover)
ISBN 978-1-250-15418-7 (ebook)

Our books may be purchased in bulk for promotional, educational,
or business use. Please contact your local bookseller or the Macmillan
Corporate and Premium Sales Department at 1-800-221-7945, extension
5442, or by e-mail at MacmillanSpecialMarkets@macmillan.com.

First Edition: September 2018

10 9 8 7 6 5 4 3 2 1

For the machines
and the people
who love them

Contents

Don't Unplug

Big Mother:
The Maternal Surveillance State

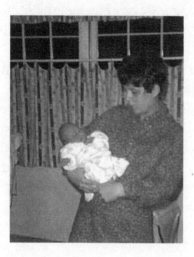

"Necessity is the mother of invention."

—English-Language Proverb

Christmas fell on a Thursday in 2003, so I had been looking forward to the long four-day weekend for a while. I knew I'd be at my favorite dive bar around the corner, the Atrium, by early afternoon. I just had to make it through the morning festivities, trying to put on a good show for Doug.

Every year, my partner, Doug, decorated the whole house for Christmas and spent hours cooking a delicious meal. But I could never work up any enthusiasm for the holiday. Every year, I swore to myself that I'd do my best, but this year was starting out just like all the rest.

I was sacked out on the couch, a 64-ounce Double Big Gulp from 7–Eleven on the table in front of me. Across the living room, my dog, Buster, was lying on the floor, looking about as healthy as I did. His eyesight was failing; he'd been diagnosed with diabetes two years ago. The vet had assured us he would live a long life as long as we gave him his insulin and watched him closely, but from what I could see, he was getting slower and slower.

"What do you think Priscilla is up to this year?" Doug asked with a sidelong glance.

Priscilla, my mother, was a distant character in my life. A few months ago, I had written her an email when I was in a particularly bad state. I just as quickly regretted telling her so much—she wanted to help, but really, how could she? She lived far away with my father, to whom I rarely spoke, and she knew nothing of my complicated world. I shrugged my shoulders and lit up my tenth cigarette of the morning.

My uncle Joe, my father's brother, would be arriving any minute. Uncle Joe was a divorcé with a few anger issues, and as he lived not far from us in Denver, he usually turned up for the holidays. I used to think it was nice of us to invite him to visit, but in reality, I probably invited him because he would inevitably start a fight, threaten me or break things. That destructive nature was familiar to me—it ran deeply in my family. His presence gave me a good excuse to go hide in the basement.

My mother, who lived in Florida, didn't usually send gifts all the way to Colorado. But this year was different. Several days ago, some carefully packed boxes had turned up at our front door. Doug, who had apparently been given explicit instructions, had been guarding them since they'd arrived. I had to admit, I was curious.

It was 8:30 a.m. All I wanted to do was smoke another cigarette or two, finish my vat of soda and go surf the internet in the safe darkness of my basement, though I suppose it was time to put some clothes on.

I descended the stairs—down to what Doug called my warren. After five years with Doug, I had finally taken my drug and internet use down to the quiet basement. I was a 35-year-old drug addict, already half-dead, with very little to show for the life I'd lived. The warren suited me just fine.

My room in the basement, what I liked to think of as my office, did look a bit like a warren. Thousands of photos, clippings and souvenirs were pinned to cork boards covering every square inch of the walls; my entire life, a story told on hundreds of pieces of paper, was displayed around me. Here was all I had seen, accomplished, lived and loved. I had the paperwork to prove it.

Buster started to bark upstairs. Shit. It was time to do Christmas. I trudged slowly upstairs again.

At 35, it shouldn't have been this hard to climb ten stairs.

"Hello Christopher!" Uncle Joe called out at top volume.

I shuffled through the living room, trying to ignore the lights, gifts and decorations Doug had hung so carefully. It was all so beautiful, it hurt to look at it. I grabbed the gifts I had wrapped for Joe and Doug and tried to hand them out—I liked giving gifts at Christmas, especially ones I could not afford. I craved the instant gratification of other people's gratitude.

"Hang on, Chris," Doug said gently. "We have a phone call to make." I sat down impatiently, but kept my mouth shut as Doug started dragging boxes out of his office where he had hidden them. My impatience turned to excitement; what was my mother up to?

Doug dialed my mom, then handed me the phone.

"Hello?"

"Hey Mom, it's Chris."

"Merry Christmas, Christopher!"

"Merry Christmas, Mom." My tone softened when I heard the excitement in her voice.

"Christopher, listen to me. Are you listening?"

"Yes, Mom." I rolled my eyes.

"I'm serious, listen to me," she said firmly.

"Ok Mom, I'm listening."

"The boxes that I sent you? You have to open them in order, ok?"

"What order? What are you talking about?"

"Open the first box and take out the book inside."

"Ok, I'll have Doug help me and then we'll call you back."

"*Christopher*, stay on the phone with me!"

Why was she so serious this morning? I smiled to myself and grabbed the first box.

"Ok Mom, I see a blue binder."

"Christopher. Now listen to me carefully. Before you open it, make sure it says 'Book 1' on the inside."

I lifted the heavily worn binder out of the box and opened it slowly. "Book 1" was written on the inside cover in thick red marker.

My mother had always had a flair for drama. I heard her exhale slowly.

"Christopher, you know I couldn't always be there with you and your broth—"

"Yeah Mom, I know, it's ok," I cut her off. She had always felt guilty about how much she'd missed when we were young, when she was busy working two or three jobs at a time to keep us from losing our home. "Don't worry, Mom, I know. And I love you."

I could feel myself getting choked up and coughed slightly to hide it.

"Christopher, I always wanted to be there for you, you know that. But just because I couldn't, that doesn't mean I wasn't keeping track of you and your brother," she said, then paused. "Ok, now go ahead and open the book."

I turned to the cover page.

> *February 17, 1968. Christopher, it's Mom, I just found out you're on your way to me.*

I knew instantly what I held in my hands. I began to sob.

"Christopher," my mom said gently. "Now stop that, Christopher. Just stop."

My mother's letters were legendary. For decades, she wrote long notes in perfect cursive to our family members abroad. Every aunt, uncle and grandparent had always talked with reverence about my mother's famous letters. I realized that this one was not just to me, but to a me that was yet to be born.

I quickly turned the pages. There was more than just one letter. My mother had, unbeknownst to me, created a time capsule of my entire childhood. Each page was numbered, dated and cataloged. Everything from my first word to my first step to my first haircut. The binders were filled with memorabilia from my childhood—report cards, my measurements, my weight, my height, notes about which foods I liked.

I began to short-circuit.

I told my mother I had to go and hung up the phone. I heard, "Christopher wait . . ." as I put the receiver down. Doug stood there looking down at me with this goofy grin on his face, and Uncle Joe smirked at me.

I had been entirely upended by my mother. She had sent me the sum total of my life to that point, catalogued, described and ordered.

A life, one that had been filled with achievements, all

slightly dimmed because my mother had mostly been missing. But after all that, she had been there. She had been there for me.

I stood up and reached for my cigarettes.

"What are you doing?" asked Doug.

I looked at him with swollen eyes.

"I'm going downstairs to my computer."

I opened the door to the basement. I could feel the numbness returning. Soon I would be safely back online, ignoring the world around me.

PART ONE

BITS AND BYTES (1968-2007)

"Everything not saved will be lost."

—Nintendo Quit Screen

I don't think that you're addicted to your iPhone, that technology is ruining your children or that Mark Zuckerberg is selling your data to the Russian government.

Nor do I think that conversations are less authentic, people are more distracted or that we are living in a simulation. (Ok, there are times I do think that maybe we are in a simulation, but that's for another book.)

So if you're looking for a guide on how to fix your life by blaming Silicon Valley, there are hundreds of resources for that online.

I do believe there are different choices you can make with the technology in your life, and maybe there are some alternative uses for the technology you hold, consume and use every day.

This book is about that choice, the choice not to become digitally Amish.

✦ ✦ ✦

I grew up partly in a small farming community in rural Maryland.

My mother would drive my brother, Chucky, and me up to Amish country in Lancaster, Pennsylvania, on the weekends. Chucky and I would eat candies made by men with long beards while Mom browsed the cookbooks and dreamed of living a simpler life.

The Amish, as I understand them, are not anti-technology. They have a level of sophistication with technology that is in line with their values and made a decision as a community that more technology wasn't needed.

Nor are the Amish like the townsfolk in *Footloose* who made rock music illegal to help keep the kids grounded in good wholesome values.

A horse, buggy, books, homes, plows, indeed everything most of us would consider necessary for glamping, or glamour camping for the uninitiated, is enough for the Amish.

But this book is about allowing progress to be progress and you to be you and finding a way to use technology to make your life better.

Rachel Hunter, the 80s supermodel, once asked me, "Do you really wear all this technology?" To which I responded, "Do you wear technology, or does technology wear you?" The choices in our life here in 2018 are really that straightforward.

We have left the time where we can safely say that we are no longer influenced by the tools and mediums around us every day.

Even if you could somehow find a way to leave the modern world, the people you interact with have been turned into de facto proxies for the technology that surrounds us.

The most significant technology hardware releases in the past two years from tech giants like Apple and Google don't even have a screen. Apple's wireless headphones have replaced screens with sensors to detect when they are in your ears and change songs when you tap them.

Devices fill our homes with music, advice, cooking timers and weather alerts. Our cars have features that block text messages while we are driving to keep us looking at the road and not our phones.

Nope, I'm not worried about a world with people who are dumbed down, looking hopelessly lost as they wander down the street with a stiff neck staring at their phone. I'm concerned about, and I would like you to be aware of, what life would be like in a world without screens where programs make decisions based on your habitual behavior.

For instance, when your devices offer you a faster way to the fast food restaurant you go to every morning to catch up on email. Or YouTube provides you more videos on terrorism after you watch one and you get the feeling you are three suggestions away from the no-fly list. Or the fact that Spotify, Netflix and Amazon know what to play, offer to show you and reorder, even when you don't know what you want yourself.

This book is a record of my journey over the past ten years. It's broken into four sections: "Data," "Information," "Knowledge" and "Wisdom." You'll read about the data I collected and what I learned. I'll then pass along some tips for your consideration.

✦ ✦ ✦

My editor often reminds me that when you write a book you have to make a promise to your readers. Here is my promise to you: To make you wiser about life in this hyper-connected, media-saturated, digitalized, streamed and downloaded culture. And to leave you profoundly more aware of who you are and what you value.

As you read this book, I want you to start to unpack your own emotions surrounding connectivity and technology. Are you holding a book right now? A real, physical book? Can you admit that it makes you feel slightly superior that you aren't on a screen? Have you surrendered to digital technology in the hopes that you are optimizing your life, health and mind, milking every second out of your day, searching for the next biohack, vitamin or software to enrich your *flow state*? Are you feverishly looking for the quote to copy and paste to your Facebook page or Twitter that summarizes the brilliance of this book, and, for that matter, how brilliant you are?

Each time you interact with software or hardware—every moment that your relationships are mediated by a piece of glass or a wireless earbud or managed by some other publicly traded entity—you have the opportunity to wake up.

Becoming digitally Amish is not really an option. And there is no prescribed length of time you could take a break from your screen that will actually make life ok again. If you think that the former tech bros in Silicon Valley—all of whom are now having second thoughts about what they have created—are going to find a way to fix this, think again.

No, this book is the only thing between dystopia and digital salvation; that is my promise to you.

You're going to learn about your digital doppelgänger, your cybernetic shadow. I'm going to help you stop valuing your schedule and start scheduling your values. You're going to learn to stop counting steps and start taking them. In the process, you will grow, learn and think differently. With my apologies to Apple, we need to move from iPhones to "wePhones." This is where that journey begins.

I can say this to you, because I didn't unplug, and neither should you.

1

Ms. Pac-Man Is a Life Lesson

To Play the Game, Learn the Pattern

Priscilla Jane Dancy gave birth to me in October 1968, the same year that DARPA, the US government's Defense Advanced Research Projects Agency, which studies advanced technologies, ordered the first router to power what you and I call the internet.

My mother was famous in our extended family for her attention to detail, handwriting and ability to walk up and down steps on her hands while smoking a Pall Mall Gold. From my mother, I inherited her undiagnosed obsessive compulsive organization.

My mother kept checklists, journals and notebooks filled with dates, facts and figures. Her organization rituals were broken into daily reviews and yearly planning. These were times where she sat down, pens, paper and index cards in hand, and asked for my assistance.

The most elaborate ritual of each year came around Thanksgiving, when my mother would go to the Hallmark store at the mall to pick up a new 18-month calendar for the upcoming year.

I would sit with her for hours over multiple days, reviewing each month of the current year, looking for special events, holidays, anniversaries and birthdays. This calendar would become the holy grail of our family's year.

My father, who kept the family in perpetual debt with his desire to purchase the latest consumer electronic or new accessory for his motorcycle, passed on to me his ability to be both the center of attention in any gathering and the most hated person after leaving the room because of his ability to articulate anyone's deepest vulnerability.

The few friends I had growing up were not allowed to visit our home. We were *that* family. The one with the unkempt lawn in a neighborhood of perfect lawns. The family with the parents that were never home yet had a driveway full of cars.

Retreating into my bedroom, I would hide out, making lists of my own, obsessively reorganizing my music and book collections and color-sorting my clothes. It was where I felt safe.

The power of being able to catalog a database of items was intoxicating, it helped me feel in control. By the time I was 14 years old, these systems of categorization and documentation could be computerized. So it came as no surprise that technology would become my next all-consuming passion.

If and when I left the house in these formative years, I headed to Blazing Flippers, where I would spend hours on Ms. Pac-Man.

Ms. Pac-Man, each ghost a different color, each color representing a different set of behaviors. Blinky, the red and most aggressive ghost, was my favorite to study.

Four different mazes, each level a brand-new prize, a colorful fruit at the center of the board that offered you the chance to gain a few extra points.

After a summer mastering Ms. Pac-Man, I was picked up by my father at the arcade one day. Lost in the music and a near-perfect game, I felt a tap on my shoulder.

"Christopher, we have to go," he said. I looked over my shoulder and was shocked to see him standing there. My father never came inside.

"Hold on, I have a nearly perfect game here!" I murmured. I could feel him gazing over my shoulder. "Damn, you're really good at this," he said.

My father, who rarely congratulated me on matters outside of physical labor, a tucked-in shirt or staying quiet when company visited, was obviously excited to see me master this game.

But outside of those carefully ordered patterns on-screen, my life was a bit more unpredictable. The summer before I entered high school, everything came crashing down around me. One night, my father asked one of his regular customers, Wanda, to close his bar so he could head out early. While closing, Wanda and her husband were shot and killed, and the bar was robbed.

A lawsuit, along with a civil action started by Wanda's family, would drive my parents into foreclosure. One afternoon, my parents called my brother and me into the kitchen and told us to pack up. There was an auctioneer at the front door. We had lost our home.

I started high school mere weeks after our move to Westminster, a small town with not much going on. My father managed to find a job working at a used car dealership. It was 1983, and this was his first job with a computer. It changed my life far more than it did his. Up until that point, I had only ever used my uncle Joe's Tandy TRS-80, and I thought my father's new computer was magical. Like any 14-year-old eager to please his dad, I was happy to help him learn how to use it.

I made frequent trips to his office to install and configure software and teach him how to input his customers into Lotus 1-2-3, a relatively simple DOS (disk operating system) spreadsheet program that defined office computing in the early 80s. My heart filled with hope just sitting down at a keyboard, even if my only task was typing "DIR," the directory command for DOS, and watching my life scroll by on the screen.

After I had finished training my father, I started visiting the dealership to work on my own projects. This computer would eventually house all the lists my mother would ever create, a place where all my memories would be collected, sorted and, most importantly, saved and recalled.

My first personal project on my dad's computer would be to build a spreadsheet of my extensive Michael Jackson memorabilia. Anyone who came to see my family between 1984 and 1988 spent quite a bit of time staring in awe at my room. Literally thousands of Michael Jackson photos, records, T-shirts and other souvenirs littered the walls, filling every nook and cranny. It looked like a museum.

Upon graduation from high school, I went off to college at Mount St. Mary's in Emmitsburg, Maryland, a Catholic university and seminary. While my parents didn't have the funds to send me, a combination of loans and grants got me in the door. There I explored Eastern philosophy and spent a lot of time reflecting on life, religion and meaning. Unfortunately, by the time the second semester came around, my mother had misused some of the funds that had been set aside for me and I was asked to leave. I was devastated. On the ride home, I stared out the window as Michael Jackson's "Man in the Mirror" played on my Walkman. How would I ever become a real adult if I didn't go to college?

College had been a safe place for me to explore and look inside myself. My family home was the opposite—never safe, never secure. But I could always find comfort in the green glow of a computer screen, in the stream of 0s and 1s running through my head in repeating and predictable patterns. On a computer I was always in control. Online I understood myself.

Several weeks after I was forced to drop out of college, my mother's best friend reached out to me. Judy ran an antiques shop in Westminster. She wanted me to set up a computer system that could track her inventory and sales. Things were looking up. I now had a paying gig as a computer consultant.

No matter how unruly my life became, I made sure my jobs always included access to machines. In September of 1992, I got my first copy of Microsoft Office for Windows 3.1. It was revolutionary!

I was finally branching out beyond the world of the spreadsheet and finding the playgrounds of word processing with Ami Pro and my first real calendar program, Lotus Organizer. I was that odd employee who carried a diskette back and forth to work so I could update my files, my calendar, even my contacts on work computers while I was on my lunch break. A cigarette in the ashtray next to me, the churning mechanical sounds of a floppy drive reading my files in front of me and a Double Big Gulp of Diet Coke—I was in my element.

Unfortunately, my unhealthy lifestyle was starting to take its toll. Between home and work, I was sitting in front of a computer for 18 hours a day. I was eating junk, indulging in as many cigarettes, as much alcohol and as many illicit substances as I could get my hands on. One Friday afternoon, shortly before diving into another weekend bender, I was sitting quietly at my desk when something snapped. It felt like my hands were not my own. I was in the middle of my first full-on panic attack.

Up until this point, there had been a few scary moments in my life where I felt afraid, but never like I was going to lose my mind. I got up from my desk and walked over to a nearby convenience store I frequented and asked John, the store manager, to help me. John, a catty old queen, probably all of 33 years old, went right into the back room, got a pill out of his drawer, put it in my mouth and locked me in the walk-in fridge.

My trips to see John to handle my panic only became more frequent over the next few months until finally, I was dependent on Xanax. This, my first dip into drug addiction, led me to finally see a shrink, who put me on the antidepressants and benzodiazepines I would take for the next 20 years.

Fortunately for me, this was also the start of me chronicling my medical symptoms in Lotus Organizer. I was patient zero in the digital health revolution—just 20 years ahead of the curve. The information I recorded in those days taught me the power of life-logging.

In 1994, I left Maryland to move in with my boyfriend, Doug, in Indiana. A couple of years after that, we resettled in Colorado, where I started working for a medical software company now known as WebMD. During this stretch of time, the consumer internet was birthed, email started becoming a necessity for anyone in business and the PC became mainstream, making Bill Gates one of tech culture's first heroes, an unlikely titan who had dropped out of college and made something of his life. (Maybe there was a chance for me after all!)

By the close of 1998, I basically lived in Microsoft Outlook, and I was copying mountains of stats and facts into my calendar each day. Years of sitting with my mother making lists had morphed into a daily and sometimes hourly relationship with software and computers. Microsoft Outlook, the flagship PIM (personal information manager), would define the next decade of my career, and I was just turning 30.

2

Do You Trust This Computer?

Your Internet History Is Still History

By the year 2000, I had backups of nearly five years of calendar entries in Microsoft Office, seven years of emails, six years of chat messages and every document I had ever created since I logged *Rock with You*, my first 45 single with a picture sleeve, in 1982. I could search my life, all of it, or at least everything I had saved thus far.

Not only that, I had a filing system that went to ridiculous extremes, folders within folders, nested by type of file or year. I could find documents to fix a problem at work from a job I had done five years earlier. I could summon an email from a decade ago. The age of weaponized facts, screenshots of conversations, saved emails and recorded conversations was still 15 years away, but I had amassed not only an arsenal but a mutually assured destruction protocol for almost everyone in my life, past, present and future. I had built the Internet of Me.

I had gone from someone who casually managed support systems at WebMD to the guy who installed the help-desk systems for the US government after 9/11 at the State Department and the Federal Aviation Administration. From FTD Florists to Einstein Bros. Bagels, from the Browning Arms Company to Blue Shield of California—if there was a help desk somewhere in the world that needed someone who understood how hundreds of connected systems, populations and processes worked, my phone rang.

But for all the extreme organization of my computer life, my *real* life was a mess. My 30-year-old body was starting to fail; I had regular panic attacks, tachycardia, blood sugar problems, insomnia and rage issues. And I was a workaholic.

✦ ✦ ✦

The shift from my life being hyper-documented to hyper-connected started quite simply. One day I couldn't find something on MySpace I knew I had posted. Have you ever had that file or post that you know, without a doubt, you created, but you can't find it? Yeah, that happens to other people, but it doesn't happen to me. Ever.

On that fateful day, I freaked out. Then I realized a fundamental flaw in my system that I hadn't planned on. The network I was posting information to was hosted by someone else, and unlike my Outlook calendar, documents and files, there was no backing up MySpace. For the first time in my life, I didn't own my own information. This wouldn't do.

Having spent years organizing files, databases and systems, I began thinking about how to construct a system that could house my life.

How would you house your life if I asked you to? Have you ever thought about your life through the lens of a computer connection?

For me, the first step was thinking of a tool I could build or use that would enable me to understand my daily habits.

More than anything, there had to be a way for it to keep track of things as they happened.

I wanted a tool that was also universally understood, searchable and had a method for defining goals. The more I thought about my requirements, the easier it was to see.

I needed a calendar.

Having spent years working with calendars, from my mother's yearly planning sessions to my 1998 MS Outlook, measuring time and data was something that came instinctively to me.

To get my data into the calendar and not spend all day in front of a screen, I had to think about a natural way to download my life online.

In 2008, the tech tool of choice for geeks was called RSS, or really simple syndication. RSS was a web protocol that allowed anyone to subscribe to a site and receive updates.

It's hard to imagine that less than ten years ago we had to basically code our browsers if we wanted news alerts.

I went to work setting up RSS feeds that would update my Google calendar every time something happened to me online.

Someone liked a Facebook post? Calendar entry. Received a work email? Another calendar entry. I sent out a tweet? Calendar entry. Listened to a song on Napster? Entry.

Within a year I could search every post I had on social media, any song I listened to and instantly see what else had happened that day.

My calendar, just like Frankenstein's monster, was coming to life.

After all my social media posts, songs I played and ranting opinions were captured inside my Google calendar, I decided there needed to be a way to see at a glance if I was spending my entire day sending emails, tweeting or watching YouTube videos. I needed to color-code my entries according to category.

Over the next two years, I would capture and catalog my spending, health and travel and even log prayers and meditation.

Imagine for a moment what your life would be like if you could open a browser, go to Google and search for "happy days." Or see days filled with red posts showing how much time you were working and see the late nights and lack of sleep that resulted.

What if you could browse your life as quickly as you could find the closest pizza joint?

That's what I could do in 2012.

I didn't stop there; a busy calendar does not transform a life.

Now imagine if you could get warnings when you're doing something that's unhealthy. Like, "Go home, you've been at the office too long," or "Stop spending money; you're at 30 percent of your credit limit."

My life had become as searchable as the internet.

✦ ✦ ✦

This book is about my search for who I was so I can help you figure out who you are—in other words, how we can use data, computers and technology to see our real selves more clearly.

I want you, the reader, to use this book as a guide to the promise of technology. Any book can focus on the everyday dystopia of technology. My ten-year journey isn't meant to be a how-to guide for you, but it is filled with many good options. Just like technology, my journey is a series of preferences configured and tweaked, saved and shared.

For all of you confused, tech-addicted, unfulfilled souls out wandering the world, seeking solace and meaning from some power higher than Steve Jobs, I wish you nothing less than full-blown digital salvation.

PART TWO

DATA
(2007-2010)

Social Media, Entertainment and Opinion

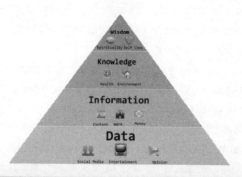

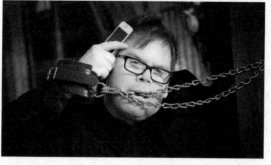

"If something is free, you're the product."

—Internet Maxim

D ata is not information. This may seem obvious to you, my savvy reader, but in a world driven by trends, clicks, page views and followers, data is king. It's the commodity for almost every business conversation I have had over the past several years. No matter what you are discussing, you can always slap down, "But the data shows . . ." or "If we had the data . . ."

Let's get something straight right now: data is simply something we use to justify our attention. In a culture where we are bombarded with things to focus on, data is all we have to filter out the noise. Think about how you process the world around you. Every piece of content you consume has been filtered by some piece of data.

We humans love to judge and think. But in an era of artificial intelligence (AI) and neural networks, judging and thinking is pretty common for computers too.

So, what truly separates humans from computers? To understand how I have learned to see the world through mountains of data, we need to first take a short trip through the complex evolutionary process of the human brain, because data only speaks to the oldest, most primitive parts of our brain.

Our brains have three distinct areas of function. Smallest and oldest, the reptilian brain controls our autopilot fight, flight or freeze responses to dangers in the environment. Have you ever seen a lizard stop to think about how much time he has left to live or where he should go hang out? Nope, lizards just react.

Thankfully our brains didn't stop there, they kept evolving. Sitting directly on top of and surrounding our little pea-sized lizard brain is the mammalian brain. It focuses on more involved decisions, emotions, habits and memories. This is kind of a big deal: our lizard brain lives in autopilot, while our mammal brain takes time to make a decision.

Sitting directly in front of our reptilian and mammalian brain is our neocortex, the pièce de résistance of brain technology, at least for now. The neocortex handles language and abstract thought; its main job is to reason or rationalize. When you think of the *you* inside you, you are thinking about your neocortex.

What does all this brain talk have to do with technology or even data? Let's imagine for a moment you're on the highway driving. Out of nowhere a vehicle suddenly merges into your lane without its blinker. You instinctively swerve and hit the brakes. Your heart rate accelerates, your breathing becomes shallow. As you realize you could have been harmed, the rage slowly starts to build and your mind is now racing. What if that person had hit you? Did you pay your car insurance? Then you rationalize and figure out how to react before you start retelling the story of your near-miss accident in your head (tens if not hundreds of versions of it).

Your reptile brain saved you by getting you out of the way when your fellow driver cut you off, then your mammal brain gave you the skills to evaluate yourself post-danger. Finally, your neocortex came back online and retold the story to help you figure out how to handle a similar situation in the future.

Today, we are not actually using all three of these brain areas as we take in new information. The mountains of information we receive in a single moment make it next to impossible to think at times, so we often reduce all decisions down to basic data.

Technology has created a world where humans would rather have the wrong answer now than the right answer in a few seconds. We value speed of processing over depth of computation. Ask yourself: How often do you select the fourth link in a Google search?

Now merge this simplified look at the human brain into your everyday use of technology. Is this Facebook post forcing you into a fight-or-flight reaction? Is a viral video thought-provoking, and do you share it with sympathy? Did you just read an inspirational quote on Pinterest that gave you pause? Did you then retell your story through the lens of this gift of wisdom?

The problem is not the mountains of data you process, nor is it a lack of filters for your information. No, our challenge is that we are using legacy software, our reptile brain, with our newest app, the neocortex. This is exactly where technology *should* swoop in to aid us. The problem is that the data presented to us every day is filtered by technology.

What does this mean for our future? Pick up a magazine or scan the headlines of the Drudge Report and you will encounter endless hand-wringing over today's trending technology topics like AI, machine learning or even neural networks. These concepts are all part of our conscious efforts to create a brand-new "machine brain."

This machine brain will own all the straight-up raw facts, dates and links, and not just your facts, dates and links, but everyone's. These new machine brains will process and evaluate billions of experiences to come up with a salient piece of *information* from all that data.

The people of Earth, with our aging, outdated brains, will soon start to surrender to machines our day-to-day evaluations, the ones we have long made by running them through all three layers of our human brains. We will be left with a lot of reactionary decisions made in the blink of an eye based on data with no context. Imagine a supercomputer operating like Donald Trump on Twitter. Scary.

Our brains and the contemplative nature of our neocortex, the hard-wiring that searches for meaning or even spirituality, is missing from today's computers. Most disturbingly, it is not being considered for the future either.

There are those investigating the possibility of coding or creating algorithms for empathy and compassion. It is time to talk seriously about that and what our needs will be. (I'd certainly rather have an AI built like the Dalai Lama than one coded from the whims of a madman with his finger on the button labeled "World Destruction.")

For now, welcome to the world of big data. Big data, for most of us, started with social media.

3

Social Media:
Social Media Is Neither

My Not-So-Safe Space

YOU ARE WHAT YOU LOG IN TO

Today, much of the once open and free web requires credentials to access pages, services and apps. Colorful buttons and logos adorn landing pages, offering us the ability to "Login with Facebook," "Login with LinkedIn" or "Login with Google." Never forget: when you log in to a site with your social media accounts, you are granting that service access to everything you value—people, ideas, places and relationships.

To understand social media and its place in our lives, we need to look at the role it plays in mediating our connections.

While I might be referred to as the world's most connected person, you are also far more connected than you may realize. Think about how many places you go on the web, on your phone and in the physical world that have access to your life and data. While your phone number is the consumer equivalent of your social security number, your social media credentials are pretty much your DNA.

My first question is straightforward: How many services, websites or apps are tied to your social media login? Social login, the technical name for the process of accessing services and apps via your social networks, goes beyond connecting us to friends, family and peers. Social login often connects us to entertainment services, institutions and devices. You have the option to log in to the streaming music service Spotify with your Facebook credentials and to log in to your Philips Hue lights with your Google login. Your Last.fm login, a service to find music, will link to your Spotify, which is already dangling off your Facebook login like a piece of spaghetti hanging from your lip. But what does this have to do with social media?

Everything, absolutely everything. I want you to stop thinking about social media as Facebook or Twitter. Social media has become the de facto standard for accessing services and life in the second decade of the twenty-first century.

Social media is how we connect, consume and share information. Sometimes we are sharing information with each other; sometimes services share information on our behalf.

Services continue to speak for us after we log out. This bartering with our life data like a cyborg-arranged marriage is continuously being updated and reviewed by our algorithmic *shadchans*. It's not nefarious or evil; sometimes it's simple, like a recruiter reviewing our profile on LinkedIn or a bot deciding to show you an advertisement for an event you might like.

Social login by its very nature asks you to define *who* you want to be at any moment. Are you a business professional using LinkedIn to find new job opportunities, or are you a casual-weekend thirtysomething looking to try out a new photo app? Maybe you allow one of these services access to your bank so it can analyze your spending.

For some of you, everything is tied to your Facebook login; for others, you may use Google. Regardless, when you choose an identity provider you are stating to the new service, "This is who I am."

Who are you, reader? Are you logging in to this book with your Facebook identity, your LinkedIn persona, maybe your Google ID?

As a system, a system in book form, I don't care, but I hope you start to think about life as defined by how you access information, because that's the first step to digital salvation.

Social networks are databases of our values at any moment, and we need to understand that we will be evaluated on those values. How you are treated is very much dependent on what the network thinks you value, or what it thinks the community values.

"Community" is an interesting term for a values database.

Before we debate the merits of Mark Zuckerberg targeting us, let us be clear what we are protecting. Social media is a portable version of you and your values. A digital doppelgänger that interacts with the internet on your behalf, even after you have logged off or left a service. Just like the pieces of snail mail that keep coming to your home for a resident that has not lived at your address in a decade, our data exhaust lingers on the web, looking for a home. Who are you online? More importantly, who are you online when you're offline?

BREAK THE INTERNET

In 2014, Kim Kardashian's posterior was on the cover of *Paper* magazine, and both Twitter and Facebook were trending with #breaktheinternet. The idea of creating an image so powerful that you could break social media has been the holy grail of marketers for nearly a decade. Long before the threat of nuclear war from a middle-of-the-night tweet was a daily possibility, the internet was run by Kim Kardashian's posterior.

The herculean task of transitioning from reality TV star to

brand influencer and internet superstar, something that even Paris Hilton couldn't manage, has been achieved by Ms. Kardashian and her family. But five years before Kim's backside broke the internet, the internet was actually broken by someone more recognizable and famous, if not nearly as influential online: Michael Jackson.

On June 25, 2009, between 2:40 p.m. and 3:15 p.m., Google reported that users of the service were experiencing difficulty accessing results and news sites. During the same period, Wikipedia saw 500 edits to a single page in less than an hour and Twitter's fail whale appeared when you logged in.

Michal Jackson had died. TMZ was reporting it and the world was searching for it. In one last moonwalk across our hearts, Michael Jackson broke the internet.

NEVERLAND

It's October 1983, and I'm fourteen years old. I'm sitting at my desk filling out a database spreadsheet on an Apple IIc I was using at the time when my mother called up: "Christopher, for God's sake, we have to leave!" I grabbed my gym bag packed with warm clothes and raced downstairs. "Do you have everything? Where is your hat?!" My mother was making sure I was going to be ok on my first overnight high school trip. "Come on, your father is in the car waiting." I had struggled with making friends in high school, but by today's standards my computer-obsessed life looks perfectly normal. When I wasn't at school, I was on my computer in my bedroom or playing Atari with my brother. Strangely enough, I wasn't labeled ADHD or screen addicted or any other modern pathology. No, I was just a kid.

As we pulled in and parked at Westminster Senior High School, I could see the yellow buses idling in the parking lot. "Wait, for God's sake, Christopher, they aren't going to leave without you." My mom lit her fourth cigarette since we'd left the house just eleven minutes ago and handed a brown paper envelope over the seat to me.

I remember being kind of shocked; my family had little to no extra money, and all the cash I made delivering newspapers on my Honda scooter usually went toward records, posters and food. "What's this?"

"Well, Christopher, your father and I are really proud of you for going on this trip; and we wanted to give you something to help you make friends, an icebreaker on your ski trip."

My mother was forever doing things like this. At the last possible moment, she usually showed up with a gift, note or card. Her sheer kindness and understanding balanced out all the cigarette smoking and swearing.

The big brown envelope had a return label on the corner reading "Office of Frank Dileo." It was addressed to "Mrs. Priscilla Dancy." The package was firm but no thicker than a schoolbook. If my mother's idea of an icebreaker with a bunch of freshmen was a schoolbook, I was going to have a tough four years at WHS.

My mother was hanging over the passenger seat like Kilroy, her hands gripping the back of the headrest. Her face looked almost manic with glee.

In the envelope was a typewritten note and another envelope with something sealed inside. The note read, "Chris, It was good talking to you and your mother. Please enjoy the photo and book." It was signed "Diana Douglas, the Office of Frank Dileo."

"Who is Frank Dileo?" I asked.

"I don't know, Christopher, what did he send you?"

I ripped open the second envelope. Inside was a black-and-white photo of Michael Jackson autographed to me, a tour program and a few other items.

For what seemed to be hours, I looked at this photo, I couldn't believe what I was holding. "Mom!" I exclaimed. I looked into her eyes and she teared up. "Those kids should think you're pretty cool now!"

"How did you get this?!" My mother, who was notorious for doing things that were borderline illegal or immoral, said: "Well, Christopher, I got a phone book from Southern California from the library, and I started calling around to find out who Michael Jackson's manager was, and I found this Frank Dileo character. Frank doesn't take phone calls but his secretary, Diana Douglas, is a real gem, so I got on the phone and pretended to be you and myself and told her you had cancer and wanted to meet Michael." Yes, this was my mother.

I jumped out of the car and raced toward the bus, gripping my Michael Jackson gifts, excited to show them off, log them in my computer when I got back and imagine a world where I got to meet Michael Jackson and feel as connected as he was to everything I loved.

✦ ✦ ✦

On June 25, 2009, at the Marriott just north of Denver, Colorado, I had just finished speaking to a small group of IT people and was heading to the lobby to have a cigarette with my coworker Robin.

My BlackBerry was going crazy in my pocket. The vibrations were obvious to everyone but me. "You going to see who needs you so badly?" Robin asked.

"Ok, sure, whatever," I said, pulling the BlackBerry out of my pocket, I had 30 messages. I opened up my first message: "OMG, Michael Jackson is dead." Next message from another friend: "Are you ok, I know how much he meant to you." Without thinking I pulled out my iPhone. Opening up Safari, I typed in "Michael Jackson" and hit enter. The first page of

Google, which usually showed up instantly, was static, like it was stuck.

I jumped on the hotel Wi-Fi and did my search again: nothing. Then I launched Twitter and looked for Michael Jackson. Hundreds then thousands of tweets filled my screen:

RIP MJ

THE KING OF POP IS GONE

WE LOVE YOU MICHAEL

My heart sank, I felt like I had been kicked in the gut. I got in my truck and drove back to my computer at home, where my internet was strong and I could be alone.

After a few hours of reading stories, I went on Facebook and changed my profile photo to a plain black square. For the next week I mourned and didn't log on to any social media. My childhood was dead.

LIVING AND DYING ONLINE

In the past we reserved our tributes to lost celebrities to the annual award show memorandum reels. Sitting around the living room it wasn't unusual to hear your auntie or uncle gasp, "Oh my goodness, was that this year?" as a Hollywood icon's name was read and still images of their 50-year career flashed on the TV. Today, and for much of the past decade, our idols, celebrities, peers, friends and family all die online.

We go online to read about life, but more often than we are comfortable acknowledging, what we find are the constant reminders of death. Our friends' profile photos are overlaid with filters representing different catastrophes.

It's not uncommon to be online friends with someone who

has passed away. Do you follow any celebrity pages of icons who no longer walk the earth, yet somehow manage to whisper their wishes through the Ouija board of Facebook? The days of unreleased records being posthumously shared with the world have been replaced by CGI reconstitutions of Hollywood celebrities. Lucasfilm digitizes every actor's face so no sequel in the Disney Star Wars franchise will be delayed by the inconvenience of a heart attack.

At some point we will be unplugged and if some in Silicon Valley have their way, we might even be uploaded, but this is not about the dystopia of dealing with the long since dead in bot form. No, this is about how we interact with the living today, knowing full well that with every post we are hard at work writing our obituary.

DO YOU REALLY WANT TO HURT ME?

By 2009, another icon of my childhood was struggling with his demons, including prostitution, drugs, inflated self-worth and jail time. Yes, this was Boy George. The makeup-wearing, gender-bending hero of my teen years in the 80s was in the middle of a career reboot. Along with Madonna and a host of other 80s global superstars, he was fighting hard to get noticed in a world that was living more online than on MTV. Eight years of iTunes had turned albums into downloadable singles, and a full-time connection to the internet in your pocket was about to turn those 99-cent singles into monthly subscriptions and billion-view videos.

Stefani Joanne Angelina Germanotta—or @ladygaga—has over 30 million followers on Twitter. Gaga, who joined Twitter in March of 2008, had converted legions of fans into little monsters, one of the first social media movements. Long before we had ice-bucket challenges, were supporting black lives or adding #metoo to our Facebook posts, our values were gaining visibility when they trended, and people were manifesting around values when they saw them becoming popular.

To this day, I'll never quite understand why Madonna, Michael Jackson, Whitney Houston, George Michael and Prince never got on the social media train when they had the chance. Maybe the idea of digitized paparazzi was more than they could take, but as a fortysomething who was super-connected by 2010, it was disappointing to watch my contemporaries be overtaken by this new breed of ephemeral digital celebrity.

Because of my unwavering dedication to mastering every piece of technology, software or hardware I encountered, I was doing something stunt-worthy at this time. I was maintaining a secret digital life—and not just one.

In 2010, I had ten Twitter accounts, two Facebook profiles and multiple blogs. Each of these digital doppelgängers had their own audience, and because of my ties to Silicon Valley, I owned a few prestigious handles on Twitter. One being perfect for an aging, boozed-up gay man. Yup, I was @thequeen. To this day, I'm sure Elizabeth had a few awkward mornings in Buckingham Palace in early 2012.

Unlike the Twitter handles I had for my career—@service sphere or my personal handle @chrisdancy—my secret accounts allowed me to engage in what today would be considered hate speech. I had multiple accounts because, at some point, I wanted to get a good job and I certainly didn't want to have an employer following me online and possibly firing me for something I said on Twitter.

Today Tim Berners-Lee, the man who invented the internet, follows me on Twitter, but back in 2009, Boy George was the crown jewel of followers for one of my secret accounts. Because we followed each other we could also have backchannel conversations.

With only a few thousand followers but tens of thousands

of scandalous headlines to his name, Boy George wanted his throne back. Watching his tweets, I couldn't help but feel sorry for him. How could he be so clueless about how Twitter worked, and why wasn't he even on Facebook? This was 2010! For God's sake, he was barred from America but not from the internet, America's new promised land.

Maybe I could do for Boy George what I couldn't do for Michael Jackson. Reach him, teach him, show him the ways of the internet.

> AUGUST 30, 2010
> OF COURSE GAGA SHOULD FOLLOW ME BUT THE
> MONSTER NEVER RESPECTS ITS CREATOR, LOOK AT
> FRANKENSTEIN! @BOYGEORGE

That was it; it was time for me to perform a digital intervention. Boy George didn't even know how to tag Lady Gaga on Twitter. How would he ever reclaim his Karma Chameleon title tweeting like an old person?

I sent a direct message to Boy George and gave him my real name. With the Twitter character limit I couldn't say much, so I typed out a letter and made a screenshot.

In the letter I gave him a step-by-step guide on how to tag users on Twitter. I encouraged him to get on Facebook and up his game. This was my only chance to help George out.

I then added the screenshot to a bit.ly link, which allowed me to track the message. I wanted to see if George would take the time to read my offer of help.

My mother might have had a phone book from LA in 1983 when she reached out to Michael Jackson, but I had Twitter.

A few seconds later I got a private message back.

COOL, THANKS, I WILL GET IN TOUCH WHEN I'M
MORE ON THE GROUND, MY EMAIL XXXXXXX@YA-
HOO.CO.UK XX!

Things were worse than I'd expected: Boy George was using Yahoo for email.

On my next trip to London, I contacted George and told
him I was in town and he invited me over to his place to hang
out.

Years went by and both Boy George and I would gain the
coveted blue checkmark on Twitter showing that we were verified users. George would finally reach almost half a million
followers, redeem his career and even reunite with the boys
from Culture Club.

Today, no one wants to head to Hollywood or desires to
record a hit album. Why bother? It's far too easy to drop a single on SoundCloud and send it to all your friends on Instagram or pay an influencer to mention you to their 50 million
YouTube subs (internet slang for subscriber). CNN will hire
you and your entire group of friends to make internet-ready
mini stories, like they did with Casey Neistat. Maybe if you
attack Nicki Minaj on Twitter in a rap lyric you'll get her attention and be the next big thing. I don't think Boy George would
make it today.

More about work, social media and life later in the book.
I promised you salvation, but first I need to get you to the digital promised land.

EDITING HISTORY

On August 27, 2007, I joined Facebook and by August 2009
I'd rejoined. From 2010 to 2013, both Chris Dancys lived on
Facebook. The original Chris Dancy, the one migrating from

MySpace, was a drunk, posting photos from the bar, talking politics and friending everyone who would have me. The second Chris Dancy was a bit more cautious, if still not a model digital citizen.

These two versions of myself along with ten different Twitter accounts and at least two different LinkedIn accounts ran my digital life from 2008 to 2012. During this four-year period, I had my share of midlife crises, highs and lows. But unlike a lot of my contemporaries I was carefully constructing different egos for myself and, more importantly, my online audience.

From the beginning I saw social media accounts *not* as conduits to friends, but as audience platforms. A natural extrovert online and native introvert offline, I found that social media did for me digitally what I never was able to do in the analog world: edit myself.

In 2008, the question I heard most often was, "Don't you think before you speak?" No, I don't think before I speak, that would take a lot of time and it certainly isn't exciting.

Yet, social media allowed me to have multiple identities who thought about their audience first, then created content—or in humanspeak, I could think before I spoke. I never thought about what to say online, I thought about which account *could* say it.

Have you ever wondered if your friends are leading double lives online? Not the traditional double lives, the ones filled with posts that are perfectly edited with the best versions of their lives on display. No, the kind of double life where they have two or more social media accounts?

Early in my career online and a few years before I was the world's most connected man, which version of Chris someone would be allowed to know was something I took very seriously.

Today, such extremes aren't necessary; new tools on popular social media platforms do that work for you.

On March 24, 2015, Facebook updated their software to introduce a new feature called On This Day. On This Day was billed as "a new way to look back at photos and memories on Facebook." In the tech community we instantly saw it as a blatant rip-off of a popular app called Timehop.

On This Day would go back exactly one year in your Facebook feed and resurface your posts like a kind of emotional time machine. If you're part of the two billion people on Earth with a Facebook account you've seen this memory clickbait in your notifications.

Somewhere between my multiple versions of my digital self and On This Day, Facebook did enhance their platform to allow users to select the privacy of their posts, create audiences and even have non-public pages. Long before Zuckerberg's software platform was a public utility, it was a tool for managing our connections and our memories.

But this is where the story of Facebook and identity gets tricky and where I want you, the reader, to pause for a second and reflect.

I, like you, have had a lot of cringe-worthy moments online. Unflattering photos, posts where I took a tough stance on something that was politically charged or a rant against some business that I would bring down with my social media prowess. Unlike you, I had a few different personas that posted these moments. If I needed an emergency shutoff valve, I could just delete that identity.

By creating On This Day, Facebook has gone into a territory that is a bit tougher to be objective about, beyond memory creation and deep into the heart of memory alteration.

Sometime in 2016, Facebook started getting complaints from users who were being reminded of really difficult times in the past, maybe the loss of a loved one, or a bad day at work or a post about an argument with a spouse. Bending to user demands, Facebook created a group referred to as Compassion at Facebook. The first change we saw to On This Day was the ability to edit your memories.

Yup, just like *Eternal Sunshine of the Spotless Mind*, the 2004 film starring Kate Winslet and Jim Carrey. After a difficult breakup, Kate goes through a procedure to delete memories from her mind. Not to be undermined, Jim goes through the same procedure. Charming, right? No pain, all gain.

By the end of 2016, you could easily go on Facebook and selectively remove anyone or any event from your On This Day feed. Facebook then took the same technology and allowed users to edit their year-end reviews and even introduced tools for couples in rough periods to take a digital break from each other.

Today, I have come to terms with my multiple online identities and just keep one set and roll the dice on social media Russian roulette. I don't edit my history, nor do I think about how to manipulate my identity.

Yet we are in the middle of raising a generation of people who see relationships through the lens of connect, follow, friend, snooze, unfollow, unfriend, block and remove from history.

If the maxim that those who do not learn history are doomed to repeat it is true, are we creating a digital Groundhog Day?

LIKED TO DEATH

August 2009, I took a pack of Marlboro Light 100s and broke them into little pieces, snapped a photo with my iPhone 3GS and logged on to my Facebook account. Smoking 40 cigarettes a day was taking its toll. I figured that sharing my latest digital resolution for health with my online community could be just the support mechanism I needed to finally quit smoking. But the reaction to my photo was not what I expected.

I received a few likes and comments, but not nearly as many as when I posted drunk or out-of-control pictures. Didn't my friends want me to be healthy? What was going on?

Carefully I started logging all the Facebook likes I got, along with the posts that garnered those digital micro-achievements. A strange pattern emerged. Friends didn't like posts that involved me getting healthy. Up early working, broken cigarettes, a brisk walk with the dog: none of those things were as popular as drugs, bars and rage.

On my forty-first birthday, I dedicated a heartfelt Facebook post to Doug, my partner at that time of almost 11 years. I was shocked to see that people, again, were not moved by this, but instead liked the nasty fight post I'd created a week later.

I was going to have to lead another type of digital life online. I was going to have to manipulate my health data to make it more clickbait-like.

✦ ✦ ✦

Mexico City in June is hot, and I mean super-hot. In the summer of 2010, I took a trip there for a conference, and from the moment I stepped off the plane, I started sweating profusely, and I didn't stop until I touched down on American soil again.

This was my first trip to a part of the world where I was a minority and couldn't speak the language, so the experience felt new, amazing and a little overwhelming. But I had a secret weapon: my iPhone. I had installed an app called Word Lens, which allowed me to scan signs, menus, anything printed, and instantly translate it into English.

My last two days in Mexico, I had a revelation. My phone was translating much of what I needed to read, so I wasn't speaking to that many people. Somehow my independence came at the cost of interacting with the locals. I switched tactics and hired a guide. But the rapt attention I had been paying to my behavior, via the logs on my phone, made putting my phone away far more difficult than I thought it would be.

My guide, Miguel, picked me up and we raced off to the outskirts of Mexico City to the Pyramid of the Sun. I tried to ignore the fact that every time I glanced down at my phone to capture the next cactus or hairless dog, Miguel got the saddest look in his eyes. It was only a few years into the social media revolution, but even a Mexican tour guide was passing judgment on the American who couldn't look up for more than a few seconds.

The Pyramid of the Sun is in the ancient Mesoamerican city of Teotihuacan. Its name means the "birthplace of the gods." The Pyramid of the Sun was built directly across from the Pyramid of the Moon and is the taller of the two monuments. Built around 200 CE, it is overflowing with mystery and history. I could sense its dark past, all the bloody sacrifices, exhausted pilgrimages and ancient ceremonies. I told my guide to wait for me, that I might be awhile, but I was heading up.

The 230 feet up to the top of the pyramid consists of approximately 248 steep steps. You could see all sorts of people hiking up the side of the pyramid: old, young, weak, strong. It's a tough climb for anyone, but in this heat and with my health, I was honestly afraid it might kill me.

My breath was labored and I was sweating profusely, but nevertheless, I launched my live stream via Ustream. Only a few minutes later, I stopped and rested with two older women who were coming down. I smiled politely but immediately looked down at my phone to launch Twitter to see if anyone else was enjoying my climb.

Eventually, I got up and started climbing again. This time

I made it approximately six more minutes before I was out of breath. My Fitbit had never seen me take so many steps in one day. (That day was the first time I had referenced my steps as justification for an activity. But it was definitely not the last.)

I realized in that moment that my climb was a physical milestone. Then the responsibility of making it to the top started weighing me down. What if people online saw that I didn't make it? What if my phone battery didn't last all the way up? What if I had a medical emergency on the side of the pyramid? A million what-ifs in my head instantly bumped against the physical reality of my body, and my heart started beating faster.

I looked around for someone to help me and saw a family headed my way.

"Hi, my name is Chris. I'm vising from Denver, and I really want to go to the top, but I don't think I can make it," I said to a teenage boy.

"Would you do me a favor and take my phone to the top and take some photos for me?" The boy looked at my brand-new iPhone and his eyes lit up. His mom looked at me sadly.

I handed them my phone and they continued their climb as I slowly walked back down to the bottom. It was a total of no more than 30 steps, but they were so much easier going down. At the bottom of the pyramid, I watched my proxy family carry my technology to the summit and snap photos of the landscape around us. Nearly an hour later, they came down and handed me my phone.

As I walked back to Miguel, swiping through the photos they had taken, it hit me: I had watched my technology make the journey that I couldn't.

Then I realized, *Shit! My Fitbit steps aren't going to match the photos.* So I took my Fitbit and edited the steps manually in the application. There, now everything lined up.

The irony of all my efforts was that when I posted the photos of me on the Pyramid of the Sun, very few people even liked them. I couldn't hide my disappointment. (I never did stop to think that perhaps because it wasn't real to me, it wasn't real to anyone else either.)

After I returned home from Mexico, I went out with friends, bar-hopping from one place to the next. Sometime the next day, I woke up to find hundreds of likes on my Facebook page. What the hell had happened? I looked and sure enough, I had posted photos of myself naked and drunk, wearing a cowboy hat.

It was clear as day. This version of me, the one I was so ashamed of, was the one my so-called friends liked better. The me that was trying to be healthier and more careful didn't interest these people at all.

PUPPET MASTER

Realizing just how much social media influenced me, I decided to conduct an experiment of my own.

Could I influence what one of my friends was wearing? Could I literally force a friend to choose a specific color or outfit?

Knowing that Facebook would send feedback to people based on what I liked, I picked a friend to experiment on and liked a photo of him in a bright red shirt. Over the next two months, I only liked him in red. It was really hard to not give feedback on certain life achievements, but if my friend wasn't wearing red, my lips were sealed.

Sure enough, my friend started wearing more red: Red shirts, jackets, shoes. Red hats, socks, ties. Slowly but surely, I was casting a digital spell. Other friends started chiming in, "You look great in that jacket!" I couldn't help but feel that I had created a digital contagion.

I took it further than that. I'm embarrassed to admit that I tried to game all of my relationships. It made me feel so powerful when I figured out how to essentially force people to find my posts by using location or emotion metadata when I posted.

Today, the idea of fake news and the conclusion that Facebook is toxic is hardly surprising. Even Facebook has released research showing the astounding effect their platform has on people. They have, supposedly, decided to throw out their strategy of monetization for a more well-rounded, well-being approach to friendships.

Slowly though, in the back of our phones, new systems of influence are spreading like a cyber H1N1. Systems that drive our health behavior, financial habits and viewing pleasures are now in charge of channeling and keeping our attention. For those of us who want to stay non-cyborg for a bit longer, we must remain ever-vigilant about who is controlling us at any given moment.

Who are you, what do you value, how do you remember your life and who are your friends? These are the questions we need to think about when we engage with social media and each other. There is no offline and online world, we are all involved in both full time.

My quest to quantify more behaviors would cause me to review how I was consuming media of all sorts. If my friends held this much power over my habits, what was my media diet doing to me?

There are hundreds of websites, books and social media gurus to help you manage your social media, so instead of going down an exhaustive list of tips to micromanage your attention, I'd like to suggest a few strategic changes in how you think about your social media moving forward.

Ultimately, for many people, social media is becoming too

much of a headache, so before you #quitfacebook, try these tips and don't unplug.

SOCIAL MEDIA TIPS

- ✦ **SEPARATE SOCIAL AND MEDIA:** View all social media services by the intent of intimacy in the connection.

- ✦ **DON'T BE DIGITALLY PROMISCUOUS:** There is no value in connecting to everything. In fact, it will probably harm you.

- ✦ **DONT BINGE-WATCH FRIENDSHIPS:** Time on Earth is short. Your friends should be supported when they need it—not when you have time.

- ✦ **BIRTHDAYS SHOULD NOT BE CLICKBAIT:** It's not a wish if everyone is making it.

- ✦ **TELL PEOPLE HOW TO CONNECT WITH YOU:** Create guidelines for yourself and your relationships on social media, then share them with everyone you meet.

SEPARATE SOCIAL AND MEDIA

View all social media services by the intent of intimacy in the connection.

When I got my first email account in the mid-1990s, I was so excited. I could manage requests and ask for help from coworkers without having to see them in person. By the time everyone with a white-collar job had an email account and we were knee-deep in the Y2K scare (the one where the media swore that all computers on Earth were going to stop working at midnight in the year 2000), I couldn't stand email.

Email had become someone else's to-do list for me. How did I go from feeling like I could handle anything over email to never wanting to see it again? The idea of digital etiquette was something we discussed a lot in the beginning, but now that everything was connected, we didn't give it a second thought. So what is good digital hygiene in relationships, even ones based solely in text?

In the 1998 romantic comedy *You've Got Mail*, Tom Hanks and Meg Ryan find love online, without realizing that they are right across the street from each other. Twenty years later, you would think we would have mastered friendship and love via digital connections, but we haven't.

When connecting with lovers, friends and peers, we need to look at the spectrum of choices and analyze the intimacy of the services. My intimacy technology stack (a word geeks use to describe all the services that make up a tool) looks something like this:

- **Facebook** is for anyone, it's a free-for-all. As someone who is slightly public because of the type of work I do, I can't block people anymore. I've tried, and it doesn't work.
- **LinkedIn** is my real-life Rolodex. If I meet someone professionally, I link to them.
- **Twitter** is where I follow things I'm interested in, both ideas and people.
- **Instagram** is where I keep people whose life I want to keep up with, but whose day-to-day adventures don't interest me.
- **Fitbit** is for people I truly care about, including family and lovers.
- **23andMe**, the internet genome service, is just for family or your physician.

It seems as if we have gotten so sloppy in our efforts to connect with people that we have forgotten about what it is we are connecting to. When we use these services, we are not connecting to people, we are connecting to people's data. You're not friending your new buddy on Facebook, you're friending your buddy's interests. You're not joining your boss's network on LinkedIn, you're subscribing to his next job hunt. You aren't following your hairdresser's life on Instagram, you are following their filter abilities and aspirational photography interests.

If we looked at our connections through the lens of the data the service is offering us, we would make better choices. Your bar friends have amazing Instagrams, but their LinkedIn life probably shouldn't be mixed in with yours.

The extreme fix: Declare social media bankruptcy and delete all your connections, friends and peers. Then, one by one, consider the data of your connection and pick the service that drives the most value to you.

The less extreme version: Choose to interact with only the people whose data fits your needs on each service, whatever those needs are. It sounds difficult, but once you start to examine your life through a data lens, you might find that things have never looked so clear.

DON'T BE DIGITALLY PROMISCUOUS

There is no value in connecting to everything. In fact, it will probably harm you.

Remember the last time you saw someone with 1,000 friends on Facebook, or who followed 100,000 people on Twitter or were connected to 10,000 people on LinkedIn? And you felt that twinge of disdain, wondering how in the world they can have that many people in their lives? Well, it's simple: they don't. To make matters worse, the hundreds of feedback loops that all those connections engender will only reinforce bad digital habits.

Few of us take the time to use our connections in a way that values both our attention span and our networks of data. Start by setting limits on the number of connections you have. Again, there is an extreme version: Declare war on your Facebook account, unfriend everyone in it and start over with just ten people. For a little while, just keep up with them. At first, you will ache a little from the lack of attention you're receiving. But the level of attention you can give ten friends will bring you unprecedented contentment.

Remove connections to everyone you have not met in person on LinkedIn and unfollow anyone who hasn't tweeted in a year or more. (Seriously, even the Twitter account for Kentucky Fried Chicken only follows 11 people. Those 11 people? 5 Spice Girls and 6 guys named Herb. The Dalai Lama doesn't follow anyone and the current president of the United States doesn't even follow himself. Be judicious.) We don't want to hurt anyone's feelings, but at the same time, the crush of humanity we are attempting to interact with online is actually crushing our souls.

Why is it that we don't look after ourselves digitally? You don't need less time looking at your phone; you need fewer people to look at on your phone. Treat each connection you have as precious. Don't just watch them live their lives from a distance. Talk to your friends on the phone or in person about things that are important to you.

DONT BINGE-WATCH FRIENDSHIPS

Time on Earth is short. Your friends should be supported when they need it—not when you have time.

There is nothing more harmful than binge-watching friendships, let alone pretending not to know what's going on the next time you meet.

During one of my many Facebook exits over the last ten years, it dawned on me why I hated who I was on Facebook.

Facebook had become a way for me to manage the time I interacted with my friends. Just like Netflix, I had started binge-watching my friends. If I hadn't heard from someone I loved in a while, no problem. I would just head to their page and catch up on their life. A friend was going through a difficult time? Turn on alerts for new posts from them. Excited over a big life event of a friend? Mark their posts "show first." What is Facebook but a nice way to DVR our love, interest or disgust?

Let's stop all that. Never look back at a friend's old posts, and never leave a breadcrumb trail for others. When our friends and loved ones are having a hard time and acting out online, send them a private message, at minimum. If you are friends with someone and they suddenly stop posting, check in with them. Changes in behavior online are easy to spot; don't lean on Facebook to keep you in the loop. Reach out.

Same goes for other services. Reviewing someone's career on LinkedIn or reading the last week of tweets is no better a gauge of who they are or what they believe in than rifling through their mailbox.

BIRTHDAYS SHOULD NOT BE CLICKBAIT
It's not a wish if everyone is making it.

Every year, the week before my birthday, my stomach slowly fills with dread. Soon enough my inbox and home screen are alight with alerts from my friends, distant relatives and family, all wishing me well ad nauseam. When I hear from people I haven't heard from in a while on my birthday, I don't feel special, I feel neglected. Who are these people and why are they showing up now?

As we all know, it's the algorithm. A machine is reminding people to interact with me and wish me well. Artificial intelligence is just a reminder system seeking control over more and more of our data. As we head into the 2020s we need to start focusing on what the machines can't do. Machines can't be endearing. (Perhaps with the exception of Teddy Ruxpin and Furby; those 80s and 90s sidekicks get me every time.)

But a heartfelt message the day before or the day after a big event is endearing. Sending a link to a song you and a friend enjoyed or a photo of you both together feels so much more honest and loving than the pre-canned GIFs that social media platforms offer to send on your behalf.

Beyond that, there are so many things we can do to celebrate our connections that the machines can't do yet. What about taking screenshots of text messages for a year and making a photo album of your conversations? Or skipping the birthday deluge for a friend and waiting until the day after to send a message: "Now that the algorithms have had their way, I want you to know, you are loved by me every day of the year!"

Instead of waiting for your partner or spouse to share a memory with you, next time you recall something, go to their social media feed and like it. Within seconds they will receive an update saying someone liked their post, and they will instantly be taken back to that post from years ago. Sometimes I like my partner's old posts on Instagram as a way of sending him a digital kiss.

Look deeply into the technology you use for your friendships and love and work, past the machine, to uncover the humanness buried inside. Be better.

TELL PEOPLE HOW TO CONNECT WITH YOU

Create guidelines for yourself and your relationships on social media, then share them with everyone you meet.

When in doubt, ask your loved ones what they want and need; better yet, tell them what you want and need.

I've successfully taken the approach of telling people what communication tools or screen-sharing services I want to use upfront. I also make it a point to ask people what they prefer when I connect with them for the first time. Take the time before you meet to ask: voice, camera or screen. There is nothing more frustrating, and potentially awkward, than being camera-ready for someone who is in a bathrobe or in a coffee shop. For friendships, it's ok to be upfront too: "I don't accept new friends on Facebook, let's start out on Instagram or Snapchat." There is no shame in stating what your digital well-being approach is.

Lack of leadership in digital manners, ethics and cybernetic virtue doesn't mean it's not important. In the 70s and 80s, we had very little leadership around food health.

Yet here we are 40 years later turning up our noses at any chicken dish that didn't live its last days in green pastures with a first name and a bath. From Whole Foods to GMO laws, the globe is having a very loud, constant and sometimes deeply irritating conversation about the food we eat.

Which begs the question, how many people became sick and died while waiting for society to take food health seriously? We don't have 40 years to wait for the digital-health talk. Our minds are rapidly being disrupted by a lack of understanding of what's happening to them.

We need someone who is willing to start a dialogue about the technology changes happening all over the world. Someone willing to take on the full-time job of our part-time attention span. We need an Oprah of the iPhone, a Jamie Oliver of the Fitbit or even a Simon Cowell of YouTube.

I'm not sure we will ever find this person, because technology moves faster than values, but until we do, I'll fill in.

4

Entertainment:
You Become What You Stream

Netflix Is a Hostage Situation

ALL YOU CAN EAT

From watching nonstop streaming TV shows and movies to listening to the never-ending gobstopper of music from Spotify, our attention has never been so relentlessly fought over by various companies. There is more entertainment to consume than there are people on Earth to consume it, and the number of creators is only growing exponentially.

I've often wondered if the promise of universal basic income isn't something that Hollywood invented so we could catch up on our Netflix queue.

The data that already exists about how we entertain ourselves is prolific and mind-boggling. Each year Netflix releases our viewing habits, shamelessly calling out data points like, "The shows that caught us cheating," meaning the shows that we watched with our family, but watched ahead when they weren't around. Or Spotify sending you how many hours of

K-pop you consumed while at the gym. Having your life's data neatly wrapped up and delivered to you each January used to be the sole responsibility of your accountant, bank or health insurance provider. Now your entertainment choices, the good ones and the questionable ones, can be packaged up and examined in much the same way.

After measuring my behavior online with friends and connections on social media, I knew I needed to examine the unseen world of digital entertainment.

As we rocket toward the end of the second decade of the twenty-first century, every major tech company has a content division, movie studios are consolidating and cinemas—full of reclining seats, waiters and nachos at 1,500 calories a serving— sit empty. Netflix has become successful because they know *exactly* what people watch and, quite simply, create more on-demand. They are using predictive modeling and, as Doritos use to say in the 1990s commercials, "Crunch all you want, we'll make more!" Music today isn't about number-one singles, or even downloads; we judge music based on the number of streams.

WHAT GOES IN MUST COME OUT

What we consume for entertainment shapes our world and our beliefs more profoundly than anything else I have measured. FOMO, the fear of missing out, is happening in entertainment as well; no matter how much we watch, there's just more and more to see! By the early part of the 2020s, Tesla and other autonomous vehicle companies will no doubt have complete content divisions churning out films to be shown inside their self-driving cars. Taylor Swift's twenty-fifth-anniversary album in ten years will be exclusively heard first in Toyota's autonomous fleets.

In 2018, MoviePass, a service that charges $10 a month and

allows you to see as many movies as you want at the theater, quickly rocketed past one million users. Anyone with a family knows you practically need a second mortgage and two incomes to see one blockbuster. It's common to spend close to $100 on dinner and a movie for a family of three. So how is MoviePass doing this so cheaply?

Unlike Netflix, MoviePass knows it is tied just to you; it's not sharable like those Netflix credentials you pass around to all your friends. MoviePass knows which theater you go to and can market to you all the time, sending trailers for movies they want you to see directly to your inbox every day. This is becoming vital to the massive Hollywood marketing industry, since in many parts of the globe you can get an assigned seat at the theater and show up right before the feature, thereby skipping all the previews. The dance between data, convenience and access to your ever-devolving attention span is driving the economy *and* many of our most unhealthy habits.

The data behind entertainment services is like a Rorschach test for cyborgs. Why is it that Spotify knows when I'm fighting with my spouse, YouTube understands when I'm depressed and Snapchat knows when I'm hungry? Simple: data. The real question you need to ask yourself is, why don't you know? And, beyond that, what could you do with the data about your consumption if you had access to it?

Once I had the data on *how* much media I was consuming, how often, how obsessively, it was clear that I was watching or listening to *something* pretty much all the time. It was time to start watching myself.

THE LIBRARY IS OPEN

I decided to look at entertainment through the lens of old and new mediums. I started with the old: books, TV and movies. Long before Netflix-and-chill streaming behaviors were the

norm, I was already spending absurd amounts of time consuming entertainment.

Binge-watching was an old behavior for me; throughout
most of the 80s and 90s, I recorded hundreds upon hundreds
of TV specials so that I could watch nonstop for hours while
fast-forwarding through the commercials. Mixtapes and an
auto-rewind feature on my boombox created analog playlists
that kept me going for an entire afternoon. Then, after multi-
disk CD players that held a hundred CDs were invented, I could
listen to a week's worth of music without lifting a finger.

Eventually, with the increasing shift to on-demand media
in the 2000s, my consumption reached new heights. While
some people were couch potatoes, I had become a TiVo spud.
TiVo, with its childlike interface, appealed to me on an almost
visceral level. All those pleasing pings and bongs and audible
clicks made me feel, for the first time, that my TV had turned
into a computer, which for me was a dream come true. Just as
the iPhone made websites superfluous, so too did the DVR
make live TV obsolete.

Yet there still wasn't a way to review what I was watching
or when. And losing productive time while binge-watching TV
was starting to become a real problem for me by 2010. *Well,
there must be an app for that*, I thought. Sure enough, after a
quick search, I found GetGlue, an app to share what you
watched on TV with your social media friends.

Basically, both GetGlue and its successor, tvtag, functioned
as a cross between Shazam, the music-identifying app, and
Foursquare, the location-based local search app. Now, when I
watched TV, the first thing I did was check in. This created a
simple dataset that allowed me to see my entertainment consumption at a very detailed level. Basically, I was about to become my own Nielsen family.

At first it was a bother to go to the TV, find my recorded

shows, and then remember to check in. But luckily my friends were doing something else I was unprepared for: they were surfing their phones while they watched TV. So while I was checking into my favorite episode of the current cultural delight, my friends were noticing my post on Facebook and answering in real time. My behavior was instantly and powerfully reinforced.

As I was trying to figure out how to track my own consumption, it became clear that soon everyone would be doing it, and it would become a matter of great importance for showrunners, TV producers and media companies. The audiences for my favorite TV shows were creating fan groups and even discussion forums to watch shows live together, albeit from the privacy of their own couches. For better or worse, I would never watch TV alone again.

GET SMART? NO.

When the data about my habits started coming in, it was pretty disturbing. At first, just seeing how late into the night I watched TV was mind-blowing. According to my data feed, I often sat down around 8 p.m. and didn't get up again till the next morning, because I usually passed out in front of the tube.

Once I had gotten over the horror of seeing my bad habits captured in hard data, after about three months of TV-logging, some subtler patterns started to emerge. First off, I had an onagain, off-again relationship with binge-watching. I would binge wildly, then go a few days with no TV consumption at all. Long gone were the days where I had a childhood ritual around which TV show I would watch on a certain day of the week: Tuesdays were *Happy Days* and Saturday mornings were *ThunderCats*. No longer did I rearrange my week around TV; now I rearranged my TV around my week.

How did the existence of on-demand change my schedule?

It was very simple: if you're going to binge-watch, just like with any other toxic binge, you plan ahead. I filled the house with the essentials—for me, Diet Coke and Marlboro Lights—and I would even clean up the basement where the 50-inch TV lived. Once my preparations were complete, I would camp out and consume.

Even though TV was now technically supposed to be on my terms, rather than the other way around, I still found myself rearranging my schedule around my TV binges. I made sure there were no meetings or important work scheduled for the day after a binge, and on the day of, I also scheduled my afternoons lightly so I could stop working early enough to get myself ready to fall into an alternate reality.

Funnily enough, none of these rituals were really obvious to me until I could see them on a calendar. We take for granted that we negotiate with time when we plan things. How often do we make plans by looking at our calendars and deciding something might be a bad day for *that*. (Perhaps we prefer doctor's appointments first thing in the morning, only on days we have no meetings. Then when the doctor we need to see has no early mornings available, we put off the healthy choice as long as possible out of convenience.) This kind of behavior tends to be unseen but it is pervasive.

With the data in front of me, I could see clearly that my TV-consumption patterns had far-reaching consequences. For example, I found that the amount of cigarettes, Diet Coke and food I consumed while watching four to ten hours of *The Tudors* also set into motion an eating frenzy the day *after* I binged that I had never noticed before.

While I was more fiercely focused on my habits than I was on my health at this point, I was already logging my food intake in yet another app. The day after a TV binge, I was consistently eating 3,500 to 4,500 calories, far more than I was consuming on other days.

DIGITAL PREPPING

I figured out that because of the planning that took place around my binge-watching sessions, I tended to delay a lot of eating the day of, in anticipation of that night's binge. After I collapsed around 2 a.m., I would sleep until noon the next day. But because I was waking up in my freshly cleaned house, I succeeded in giving myself a false sense of accomplishment, so I spent a lot of time the next day eating.

Yes. One of the most trenchant and frustrating behaviors I discovered over my years of self-hacking was my persistent habit of rewarding myself for good behavior with overindulging in my bad habits, in all categories.

While I always ate unhealthily, I saw that I was practically consuming straight garbage on post-binge days. I was stressed out at falling behind, having spent so much time in front of my TV, but because things around me looked as if they were technically in order, I felt justified in giving myself yet another reprieve from doing something better with my time. But 4,000 calories later, I would inevitably be filled with regret over all my choices over the past 24 hours.

I had verified something I had long believed was true: I was a consumption-aholic. All those AA meetings I had tried to go to for so many years—what a waste! If only the scope had been a bit larger, I would have completely understood why I was there and felt I truly belonged. Oh, to get back all those hours and actually gain something from them. "Hi, I'm Chris, and I'm a consumption-aholic."

By 2011, I understood that if a substance or situation could be abused, I would find a way to do so. Furthermore, if it was easy, I was very adept at finding a way to make it even easier. Maybe technology mainly serves as a constant reminder of possibilities to the craving mind?

Nowadays, if something seems too easy, I look at it as a warning sign. Think about your life and think about how often you're frustrated. It is almost always tied to the lack of speedy access to something you want to consume. If there is one true evil in the world, it might well be ease of use and our resultant expectations that nothing should ever be difficult again.

My understanding about TV as a shared medium clarified to me how it could change my friendships without me even noticing. If I had a friend who was into the same show as me, our conversations, not surprisingly, were frequently tied to our understanding of that show. Obvious, right? Yet the 15 minutes you've spent talking about a TV show are a lost opportunity to talk about your happiness, your health, the rest of your life. It's insidious how sharing our bemusements can turn into a way to hide from ourselves, to hide behind media consumption and other people's ideas.

Next, I started looking at everything that I listened to or watched through the lens of applications. Books were probably the next easiest thing to quantify. As a child, I had always loved books, yet books had also always been challenging for me. I had trouble focusing and reading out loud was terror-inducing. But audiobooks allowed me to consume books without getting bogged down by my fear of them, so I had started listening a lot.

BOOKS AT NIGHT FOR BETTER SLEEP

Audible, the audio bookstore and the accompanying app, allowed me to take my love of learning and collecting new information to a higher level. Like most of the generation of

applications hitting the App Store in the 2010s, Audible gave
me the ability to earn badges, share my books via social media and even take notes or highlight sections within the apps.
These features then turned into a bevy of insights about my
reading habits and my journey through a book. In a few short
months, I had consumed countless books on workplace etiquette, how to speak in public and anything else that fascinated me at that moment. As I cycled through topics my tastes
evolved. I started in on history books, then tomes on Eastern
philosophy.

Did I somehow teach myself to get into books? For me, just
the act of understanding my consumption proclivity made this
next hack even easier. While I noticed that I was consuming a
lot of books before bedtime, my data also pointed to the fact
that I was using my phone at the same time. I had to learn to
separate these events in order to eventually improve my sleep
habits. But how could I log my book session on social media
without alerting my friends and getting a ton of responses right
before bed?

My solution might sound crazy, but it made perfect sense
to me. I created a series of fake Twitter accounts and tied them
to all my app-based activities. Reading a book? Tweet it to no
one. Listening to a song? Tweet it. (Room temperature change?
Tweet it. @dancyair still lives on Twitter somewhere, with the
measurements of the air quality of my home stuck back in
2013.)

Now that all my TV and book consumption was being
logged, it was time to tackle the rest of the entertainment jug-
gernaut. What about YouTube videos, movies at the theater,
podcasts and TED talks? My behavior was evolving, and my
data trackers were paying attention. Liking videos on YouTube
gave me access to the data I craved—which YouTube videos
was I watching, how often, when and how did they make me

feel? I created more and more fake Twitter accounts to track everything I saw. @dancyentertain filled up with TV, movies and all other types of content I consumed in 2012.

It sounds incredibly complicated, but in reality, once my system was set up, it was easy to track everything. And it was well worth it. I could see my behavior and how it changed before and after watching a movie. Furthermore, I could actually tell how the location and who I was with affected me.

OPENING NIGHTS ARE NOT WORTH IT

For example, I'm a big opening weekend kind of movie watcher, and because I'm also the kind of person who dislikes a bad seat, I always had to be early. That meant my entire day got rearranged to get things done faster and earlier so I could get to the theater on time. Perhaps not surprisingly, it also meant eating more at the theater. Friday night opening weekend movie trips would always turn into a disaster for my diet and exercise routines. Those Friday movies always meant moving less the day of and overdoing it the day after to try to make up for my slacking off. (After all, when you become a mere number, you will do almost anything to meet that number.)

Now aware of the wider costs of going to opening nights, I moved those showings to times that didn't obliterate my day and throw the rest of my life into low-level chaos. Moving the same movie to the middle of the day, away from crowds, or even paying more for assigned seating were simple ways I could hack my behavior to achieve a better result. I could watch just as many movies, but in this way, I regretted them a lot less.

MUSIC AND ME

Next up? My lifelong obsession: music. Did you ever have a tight deadline or maybe procrastinate too long finishing a project? Fall in love? Get dumped? Lose someone you love? No matter what, long before there was an app for that, there was a song for that. Music has always been a remarkable way to influence behavior. Like so many people, my lifelong relationship with music is the longest and deepest one in my life.

Back in the early 1980s, while most of my friends were hanging out on a Friday night listening to cassette tapes, I might have been sitting at my father's office computer, logging music into Lotus 1-2-3. I discovered a profound satisfaction in seeing my music collection organized in alphabetical order on my shelf. But with a spreadsheet, that satisfaction was eclipsed by my thrill at being able to re-sort my collection by genre, artist, album title and release date.

Fast-forward 30 years: the first time I saw my musical life perfectly ordered inside an iTunes catalog, I nearly cried with joy. We've come even further now that the world's soundtrack is an always-on AI-generated mood playlist on Spotify.

I decided to look at music consumption in two ways: passive and active. Active consumption of music meant that I decided to play something, usually when I was working or cooking. But I wanted to understand if passive consumption of music was influencing me just as much.

Passive music is harder to quantify and examine—it fills so many places in our lives, from the high-power speakers of the lowrider stopped at a traffic light next to us flooding our airtight windows with bass to the *Oh, shoot, what song is that?* feeling you get when you're standing in line at the grocery store. Our lives are filled with other people's playlists. Yet so much of this influence is invisible until that song or moment comes back to us in the form of a playlist suggestion or a reordering of our Discover Weekly on Spotify.

If Spotify or Apple Music understands enough about me to offer me breakup songs when my boyfriend and I are fighting, shouldn't it also be able to offer me a mood booster when

I'm feeling low? More importantly, how can I see those drivers and influence them myself? Is there a way to create a musical inoculation against behaviors like procrastination, fatigue and poor diet choices?

That became my mission. To get there I had to log all those songs, the beats per minute, the genres, singers and titles. But the musical consumption landscape wasn't great back in 2012; while there was a lot to listen to, there was no easy way to keep track of everything you were hearing. Until I found a service that did just that.

Last.fm was founded in 2002, as the last remnants of Napster, the revolutionary music-sharing service, were being removed by Apple and iTunes. Last.fm had a unique feature made for someone like me: scrobbling. Last.fm's scrobbling was simply a service that recorded every song you listened to and the order in which you consumed them—basically a transcript for your jams. The songs Last.fm offered me felt as magical as Pandora had felt the first time I experienced that digital DJ a couple years earlier. More importantly, Last.fm would plug right into my music habits.

Each time I listened to a song, the song, track, album and artist would be instantly saved in the order that I played them. A breadcrumb trail of what guided me through the day.

It goes without saying that Spotify, which took Europe by storm in the early 2010s from their command post in Stockholm, Sweden, was like nothing I had seen in my life. All the world's music streaming, all the time, no need to buy anything, and a never-ending list of things to consume. Luckily, Last.fm was a simple integration into Spotify. Anything I was listening to was instantly shared on Facebook and sent to my Google calendar to be categorized and tracked.

FOCUSED BEATS

My calendar exploded once again. Real-time music filled my days with hundreds and hundreds of entries. Once I could see the music I was listening to, I had a profound insight: active listening to music in 2012 meant I was stationary. I had not yet entered into the world of exercise in any meaningful way, so a day filled with music on my calendar often meant an entire day spent in front of the computer, in the car or on a plane. How could I use music to make me be more active?

Baby steps, baby steps, I thought. At nearly 300 pounds, I wasn't going to pick up long-distance running. So I started with something tangible. If I was going to be sitting, could I do something more useful with my ears and eyes? Was there certain music that at least could bolster my propensity to work and get stuff done? We all have heard of playlists that push you through that last mile in a marathon, but could such a thing exist for procrastination?

In 2012, the playlist scene on Spotify wasn't at the point where we could browse "Brain Food" or "Focus" and find songs created just for paying attention to the current task. I had to be a bit more inventive. I looked for distracting songs and started playing them while I was wasting time. Yes, I actually created playlists to listen to when I decided to wander off the path of enlightenment by opening up yet another distraction tab on my browser. The simple act of not allowing my ears a break, forcing them to listen to very distracting songs while I was distracted myself, actually started to condition me to spend less time in the timeless voids of web searches. My musical choices could in fact help me start to focus on getting stuff done.

While this path would eventually lead me into the

neuroscience of isochoric and binaural beats, in the beginning, it was as simple as finding songs that were tuned to a certain number of beats per minute, otherwise known as tempo. No one told me raves had actually been group therapy sessions back in the day. I found that music with a tempo between 60 and 80 beats per minute, basically a walking pace, helped me focus on the task at hand. Anything faster, I got distracted. When the beat was slower, I got lost or bored.

In the beginning, having my music saved as I listened to it allowed me to go back and research the music in-depth. I could find out what really motivated me or, more specifically, the music I was listening to while motivated. The formula for productivity is relatively easy. You need to look at focused effort + output. If I could figure out what music led to an increase of those two things, I could build a playlist for life.

For me, the type of work I did—usually in Microsoft Office tools: Word, PowerPoint, Outlook—was key, and an application like RescueTime, which measured my tool usage, was essential.

We all know that focused attention in a world of distraction is increasingly difficult.

As I created documents, PowerPoint presentations, blogs and even scheduled tweets, I would go back and look for clues as to whether my attention was focused. Unfortunately, I found that little to no movement helped: a day with a low step count was going to be a productive day, or on the flip side, a complete blow-off day.

Next up was location: Was I someplace where I tended to be active or stationary? Then I looked at how much time I spent in specific apps. For me, spending too much time in calendaring or email was non-focused time.

I started to string together a behavior map:

- Low steps + at work + in meetings = nothing productive accomplished.
- High steps + at work + no meetings + majority of time spent in a browser or on email = nothing productive accomplished.
- Regular steps 3,000 to 5,000 + no meetings + no email, calendar or task apps + MS Word or PowerPoint for 30 to 50 percent of my day = yup, I got a lot done.

Now, you might say, "Of course you'd get more done on a day with no distractions." But on the other hand, I now knew how to create the optimal situation for being highly productive.

This next step is easier than it sounds: get used to playing music, nature sounds or something in the background while you are working. This soundtrack will become more essential the more you listen to it as you retrain your brain to understand how to get back to work.

GO WITH THE FLOW

A goal for every life hacker is the holy state of *flow*. Flow is that feeling you get when there is nothing in your mind but your purpose and your unwavering focus. Those moments where you can feel yourself creating your future, coauthoring your destiny—that is flow. Books, webinars, podcasts, lifestyle gurus and biohackers will all give you advice for achieving and maintaining flow.

For me, flow became a delicate balance between just enough time to get something done and the conditions to get it done. Time is never really the challenge for us, although it's often the first thing we blame when stuff doesn't get done. No, for me, and for you, *conditions* are the challenge. Have you ever stopped to examine your mind when you're procrastinating? What is the story you're telling yourself?

Chances are, your mind is scanning for the "right" conditions for the task at hand. The Greeks called this *kairos*. Kairos was a type of time, a non-ordered description of when the opportune time was at hand. Temperature, light, mood, the intensity of the crowd, etc. One of the few conditions we can manipulate, control, measure and maintain is sound, and music is the surest way to create a flow state.

Learning to passively capture what you listen to while working when you're in flow is a surefire way to train your brain to go into flow with less friction next time you are facing a deadline or obstacle.

Essentially, you create the conditions for flow. Maybe it is a particular coffee shop, a particular time of the morning, a feeling before a big meal? Who knows, but your flow entry point is uniquely yours. Now, if my editor asks me for the next chapter, no problem, I have a playlist, and there is an Espresso House on every corner in Stockholm.

In the beginning I had a long playlist of old music I loved, but I found that familiar music became a distraction for me. I would be in a good flow and then a specific song would come on. Before I knew it, I was switching screens to tell my friend Sam, "Gurl, do you remember when we were at Numbers and I was twerking to 'This Time I Know It's for Real' by Donna Summer, https://open.spotify.com/track/6ez4yXpLini3DSbaLR10qZ?"

So if old tracks weren't working for me, what would? The answer came one day when I was browsing Spotify and I ran across the Discovery section. When I settled down to work, I would play anything I found on Spotify, then once I noticed I was in a flow state, I would switch the playlist over to one of these Discovery stations, thereby training my brain to be focused whenever these new tracks were playing. In essence, something I had not heard before became catnip for my distracted brain; meanwhile, my focused brain could get work done.

The conditioning pre-step was complete. Now, when I needed to focus, I'd press play on one of these playlists *hours* before I needed to start to work. The music would get my focused brain ready to slip away into a corner of a coffee shop and start to crank out projects while my distracted brain was tied up enjoying itself. Basically, my brain needed to be trained to run two processes. (This might sound kind of crazy, but it is actually related to a field of study in neuroscience called executive function.)

As I started to finally understand how all the active music I was listening to affected my behavior, I knew I also needed to capture the passive music all around me. How could I even begin to analyze its effect on me?

Then I discovered the magic of an app called Shazam. There is even a TV show now with Jamie Foxx called *Beat Shazam*; it's like *Name That Tune* meets your iPhone. But when I first discovered it, and what it could do for my quest, it changed everything. If you paid up for Shazam Pro, there was even a feature that would run Shazam in the background full time. This meant I could create a playlist from my whole day, each and every day.

This development had a profound effect on how I came to understand noise and its intense effects on my diet, activity and lifestyle. At the most basic level, there is a lot of magic in how we interact passively with the world around us. These days, I use Shazam mainly to collect music while on vacation. In this way, I can capture the tunes I hear in Paris, Barcelona or Venice and turn them into a playlist. Long after I've returned to the drudgery of the office, I can simply play my curated

"European Vacation" playlist to bring myself back to the magic of that amazing trip.

You see, your entertainment data isn't just background noise or gym motivation, it's the code for reprogramming everything you do and feel.

The rest of your life is going to be filled with content— videos, music and books that you consume passively and actively. Sometimes you will seek it out, more often than not, the content will seek you out. There is so much more to hear, see and consume, more now than ever, don't unplug.

ENTERTAINMENT TIPS

✦ **HOW THE SAME OLD SONG IS HOLDING YOU BACK:** From procrastination to new habits, your entertainment could be holding you back.

✦ **SAVE FOR LATER:** How content bookmarks work against us.

✦ **SPEED-READING:** Digital audio, video and books can be slowed or sped up. Experiment with playback speed to tune your focus.

✦ **READING YOUR EMOTIONAL UTILITY BILL:** Explore your personal trends to find moments of peace and joy.

HOW THE SAME OLD SONG IS HOLDING YOU BACK

From procrastination to new habits, your entertainment could be holding you back.

Music services, such as Spotify, Apple Music and Amazon Prime, much like social media, have a single mission: to keep you coming back. Time spent in app, which is Silicon Valley's way of saying they own you, is something we shouldn't take for granted.

If you are struggling with procrastination or challenged with any type of daunting task, just try it: listen to music that you wouldn't normally find appealing. If you can get through the first few moments, your pattern-matching mind will be so confused, you will be able to start and finish just about anything.

The second thing this accomplishes is also, in my opinion, vital: engaging in random media creates a distraction for the services.

Think of the machine algorithms watching you and serving you information, entertainment, directions as that overly eager acquaintance who wants to be your best friend. He just wants to help, but he doesn't really understand you or what you want, he just knows that each time you do XYZ, you usually want PQM as a result.

Think about how often you purposefully or accidentally distract the systems in your life. Everyone does it in one way or another. Some people type super-fast in the Google search bar so they won't be influenced by the type-ahead feature. Or maybe you let other people borrow your Netflix login or make playlists on your Spotify account.

Remember: our eager friends, the software algorithms, have only one real skill—speed. They don't know what's *right* for you, they only know what's *right now* for you.

Distracting these systems is a way to not only train ourselves to expect more from our tech but also to help prepare us for the future that newer, bigger, scarier AI will soon be bringing into our lives.

Just as Jaron Lanier wrote "You are not a gadget," I want you to remember that you are not a *habit*.

The power of your preferences *not* being saved or tracked, or better yet someone else's preferences, can't be underestimated.

I've often said that you don't need couples therapy, you just need to listen to your partner's playlist.

SAVE FOR LATER
How content bookmarks work against us.

YouTube has this neat little option called "Watch Later." But these later lists are not bookmarks, they are breadcrumb trails for your moods and interests, and they are rife with information. When we save a video for later, in essence we are saying, "I might like this, but I don't have time to invest in my whims right now." Popular web browsers and content apps also do this: Safari has an option to "Add to Reading List," and the *New York Times* app has a "Save for Later" button.

Services are watching carefully to see what you do consume, and I can almost guarantee that services also look at what you mark to read later. And if you never do read it, it is quite probable that the service will be unlikely to show you that type of data again. The opposite end of the spectrum is when we become ideologically radicalized because of how we consume media, something Zeynep Tufekci, a techno-sociologist, has written about as an alarming trend in the era of algorithmic content recommendations.

Furthermore, buckets filled with things you want to read but haven't yet will only serve to depress you. They are a constant reminder of the world you are missing out on: entertainment FOMO. Instead, try thinking of the save-for-later function as a mood marker. When saving an article, video or photo, consider it a statement on what you were feeling at that time. Furthermore, treat it like a passive diary of your life and interests. So many people today will publish a list of books they've read or songs they've consumed, yet the real value is in publishing a list, even if only to yourself, of what you wished to read but didn't.

Taking a moment to look at your entertainment to-do lists can be a real eye-opener. Look at each piece of content and think about what makes you want to keep it there. Why do you feel the need to fill your time with stuff to do? You may find that your to-do list should be replaced with a "to-don't" list.

Is it time to call entertainment bankruptcy and delete these lists?

SPEED-READING

Digital audio, video and books can be slowed or sped up.

Experiment with playback speed to tune your focus.

There are a few ways you can use data to consume more while doing less work, and I'm only slightly ashamed to share them with you.

Have you ever thought about having strangers read books to you? Well, not really, but close enough if you listen to audiobooks.

My experience with audiobooks, as you know, helped me understand a lot about my own attention and desires. But audiobooks do something else that print and ebooks can't do. They speed up and slow down. You play audiobooks at double, triple or even quadruple speed—better yet, you play the books at half speed.

While it's not a good idea to consume all your media like this, studying playback speed does serve as an interesting bit of brain science. Double-speed audio is actually a great way to get more out of a book; you'll quickly find that by listening to books at double speed, you actually pay more attention to them. All this information coming at us at twice the normal speed forces our brain to focus on what is being said. You'll consume your book in half the time, and I'm willing to bet you'll actually retain more.

Why on Earth would you slow a book down though?

Interestingly enough, listening to books at half speed is a great way to fall asleep. Your mind will slowly drift off as the speed of your internal monologue starts to match the dialogue of the slower book. There are very few times in this book where I will advocate you messing with your senses as profoundly as I am here, but I truly believe that you can master your content overload by using your attention and time to get the most out of what technology has to offer.

READING YOUR EMOTIONAL UTILITY BILL
Explore your personal trends to find moments of peace and joy.

What is so compelling about pushing all your media through digital channels and what should you take away from this chapter? Well, that depends on how much you want to learn about yourself. I like to call digital media usage my "emotional utility bill."

Just like regular utility bills, once a month or sometimes quarterly our media service providers will send us lists of what we consumed, how much time we invested in those activities and how they compare to others.

We don't often see our trends through the lens of how we are changing and evolving, but there is no reason we can't. Are you listening to more or less music? Often dips in music consumption signal life changes. How did this fall's binge-watching compare to last fall? Are those few extra pounds we put on this holiday season actually a result of our viewing habits rather than all those holiday parties? Maybe you want to change some of your own less-than-desirable behaviors or start some new rituals and retire a few old standbys that no longer serve you.

An emotional utility bill in the form of your statistics and consumption habits holds the secrets to your mood, attitude and productivity!

Next time you decide on a new show to watch, a trendy

playlist to subscribe to, or even what film to watch at the cinema, you will hopefully start to see how the behaviors behind these activities tell a larger story about you, your habits and your direction in life. You are what you eat, and you become what entertains you.

5

Opinion:
Yelp Made Me an Asshole

The Internet Doesn't Make You Right

YOUR FEEDBACK IS VALUABLE, SOMETIMES

Have you ever left a scathing review for a business, shot a video of bad customer service with the intention of posting it somewhere or marked a room on Airbnb with one star? The benefit and burden of being super-connected is no longer just how we find each other. It has quickly become how we evaluate and judge the world around us. I really wanted to understand why and how I offered advice to others, and why it was often *so* negative.

The problem comes from the awkwardly inverse relationship created when businesses stalk us for our feedback, tell us they value our opinions and plead with us to take just two minutes to fill out a survey. Meanwhile, our sense of the value of our own time is also being threaded through the eye of an ever-narrowing needle, where our deflated attention span meets our inflated digital ego.

Online data and behavior metrics will shape much of what

we see online and are offered in real life. Until the day we have Orwellian AI, our opinions of services will drive how businesses make a lot of their decisions, as well as what we ultimately think of ourselves.

Long before we had systems to provide feedback on, such as Yelp, Facebook or Foursquare, loyalty programs and their incentives drove many consumers. Your Walgreens value points and your airline loyalty miles were the golden keys to the kingdom of data. Customer satisfaction, also important, was the real-time satisfaction you had with a product or service, one that was captured after a transaction ended. Businesses pay attention to that too.

Yet it's not just transaction data businesses want from us today; no they want to know what happens after we leave the premises, abandon that digital shopping cart or get distracted by some other piece of digital eye candy.

Look at the attention to detail some of the largest e-commerce chains have put in place for after you check out. They provide a link to track your package and when your package arrives, you receive a text message. The anticipation builds and builds even if, often enough, the wrapping is more exciting than the goods inside.

So, on the one hand, we are being groomed to treat all digital experiences as events that we are encouraged to record, share and talk about. On the other hand, businesses are shaking in their boots that a poor social media campaign or transaction will go belly up with an influencer.

We are both valued and feared for our influence in today's hyper-connected retail economy. At the first sign of trouble in a retail transaction, cell phones are pulled out, videos are rolling and live streams are initiated. Social media, influence and the cult of the customer has created a mob mentality that is frankly good for business but bad for our emotional health.

OLD YELPER

I was succeeding in checking things off my self-knowledge to-do list, such as teaching my social media to start to respect me and learning how to avoid binge-watching *Dexter* or old seasons of *Lost*. Now I needed to uncover what it was that drove me to share my ideas and opinions, often negative ones, in such public ways.

From 2010 to 2015, using only my cell phone and a lot of misplaced anger, I probably tried to take down more careers than anyone I know. Everything was affecting me negatively, or at least it seemed so at the time, and I developed the addictive habit of venting online.

There was no platform that was immune from my criticism, though Yelp tended to be my weapon of choice. Even just reading the reviews and the feedback from Yelp reviews helped me understand fundamental things about the power of connected commerce.

What did it mean that I got my kicks voting up negative reviews of businesses that didn't live up to my expectations of their service? I was becoming a world-class digital asshole.

Using social media as small claims court for bad customer service was more than just a passing phase; it was an intense part of my life. Somewhere between Facebook and Yelp in 2010, I started actively reviewing business. In the beginning, it was just a fun little game—with each check-in and review, I could unlock a new level of achievement, making my reviews more important to the people who would discover me and my digital exhaust fumes on social media. Long before services like Klout were actively putting me in front of employers, influencers and the market, these online hubs for main street America were shaping me. More often than not, though, I was being shaped into a monster.

JANUARY 23, 2010: GUNTHER TOODY'S, DENVER, CO: TWO STARS: "USED TO BE AMAZING BACK IN 2004. FOOD AND STAFF ARE HIT OR MISS NOW."

While this review seems innocent enough, the response to it gave me pause. A few days after the post went up online, my phone rang. It was a manager from Gunther Toody's, asking me for more information about my dining experiences. I was blown away. Were people at this business actually reading my feedback?

A dangerous period of experimentation began. I started posting more and more over-the-top reviews, sophomoric in their comedy and outrageous in their candor. I was dabbling in the dark arts of online manipulation. And it was intoxicating.

Early in 2013, the dry cleaner I had been using for years lost my clothes. I took to the internet like Donald Trump at 2 a.m. after watching Rachel Maddow.

JANUARY 2, 2013: DEPENDABLE CLEANERS: THREE STARS: GOOD CLEANER WITH A FEW ISSUES THAT BECAME DEAL BREAKERS. I NOTICED OVER THE PAST FIVE YEARS, THE CLEANERS AT THIS LOCA-TION KEPT INVESTING IN HIGH-TECH GADGETS AND THEIR PRICES WERE NOT THE BEST. THE MOST DIFFICULT PART ABOUT DEALING WITH THIS CLEANER WAS THE CONSTANT MISSING CLOTHING. I WOULD GET BACK CLOTHES THAT WERE EXACT IN "BRAND" AND "SIZE" BUT NOT MY CLOTHES. THE STAFF IS VERY FRIENDLY, BUT THE OWNER-SHIP SEEMS TO BE LOST ON QUALITY AND CUS-TOMER SERVICE. WE DON'T NEED FLAT-SCREEN TV'S, WE NEED OUR CLOTHES OR A MORE ACCU-RATE SYSTEM. GOOD: AFTER-HOURS DROP OFF / FRIENDLY HELP / GOOD LOCATION. POOR: PRICES

/ INFRASTRUCTURE UPGRADES ARE OVER THE TOP
/ SWITCHING OUT CLOTHES.

Within an hour, Steven Toltz, the president of Dependable Cleaners, had reached out to me on Yelp.

> I APPRECIATE YOUR COMMENTS AND SUGGES-
> TIONS. I'D LIKE TO LEARN ABOUT THE PROBLEM
> YOU EXPERIENCED. WHILE IT SOUNDS LIKE IT MUST
> HAVE BEEN WORKED OUT IN THE END, OUR GOAL
> IS TO GIVE YOU READY-TO-WEAR CLOTHES EACH
> AND EVERY TIME SO YOU CAN PACK FOR A TRIP
> AND FEEL CONFIDENT ABOUT WHAT YOU BROUGHT
> WITHOUT HAVING TO LOOK. I CAN HELP WITH
> DISCOUNTS AS WELL. PLEASE GIVE ME A CALL AT
> 303-777-2673. THANKS FOR THE REVIEW. STEVEN
> TOLTZ, PRESIDENT

This was amazing. After talking with Toltz, I edited my response:

> EDIT: I RECEIVED CONTACT FROM THE BUSINESS,
> WHO WENT OUT OF THEIR WAY TO HELP ME. THANK
> YOU DEPENDABLE! NET/NET, I WOULD RECOMMEND
> THIS CLEANER.

I felt like the Yelp Hulk, green and huge and angry and ready to lay waste to anyone who got in my way. If I started leaving really positive reviews, ones that were more intimate with a social message, could I become the cyborg Ralph Nader?

> JANUARY 2, 2013: PARK HILL DRY CLEANERS: FIVE
> STARS: HAVE BEEN USING THIS CLEANER FOR ABOUT

FIVE MONTHS NOW, SINCE SWITCHING FROM DE-
PENDABLE CLEANERS IN CHERRY CREEK . . . WHAT
I FOUND, A FAMILY RUN CLEANER . . . EACH AND
EVERY VISIT, I'M GREETED WITH MY NAME AND
ALL MY CLOTHES ARE CARRIED OUT TO MY CAR.
THE PRICES ARE HALF OF WHAT I WAS PAYING, SO
I NOW DO MORE DRY CLEANING AND LAUNDRY
THAN I EVER HAVE IN MY LIFE. THE VALUE OF THE
RELATIONSHIP THAT THIS SMALL BUSINESS HAS
CREATED WITH ME IS AMAZING. I LIVE IN PARK
HILL, SO SUPPORTING THE LOCAL BUSINESS, AS
WELL AS SUPERIOR CUSTOMER CARE, SEEMS LIKE
A WIN—WIN. YOU CAN'T GO WRONG HERE, SLOW
DOWN AND PUT YOUR MONEY BACK IN THE COM-
MUNITY AND EXPECT QUALITY.

Within three days, my glowing review had garnered 13 useful votes. While I had not been loyal to my first dry cleaner, being
a nicer customer online actually garnered me more attention.

But my kinder, gentler self was constantly overshadowed
by the angriest version of me. My reviews and tweet storms
were becoming darker, the feedback loop was getting faster and
the possibility of one of my posts going viral, and me wanting
to be able to back up my stories with mountains of proof, was
driving me to weaponize more and more data about my experiences. What if I included my heart rate, my bad night of sleep
and the fat and sugar contents of a meal in my reviews?

TOO MANY BAD REVIEWS AND YOU'LL NEED AN ANTIDEPRESSANT

The internet made everything go faster, especially hate. I had
discovered a Moore's law for emotional health. Moore's law, the
computing paradigm coined by Gordon Moore, states that the
"number of transistors in a dense integrated circuit doubles

approximately every two years." (It's a common trope. There is even a Zuckerberg's law, named after Mark Zuckerberg of Facebook, which states that people share twice as much each year as they did the year before.)

For me, at the point where Moore's law met Zuckerberg's law, there was a cyclone of depression and self-loathing. I knew I had to rein in my inner asshole. I needed to better understand what was going on when I shared my opinion. There was clearly a well-worn path I was treading before spewing my venom online:

1. Feel entitled: I deserve to be me, unedited.
2. Spend money: The world is mine and I'll pay this bill off someday.
3. Find someone else and make them have a bad day to make yourself feel bigger or better: Forget other people are human and expect them, at minimum wage, to treat you like royalty.
4. Post and shame: Get someone fired and teach the world who they are dealing with.
5. Tell all your friends and then fight with them when they point out valid concerns for others: Why can't you see my pain? Fine, I'll block you on Facebook.
6. Stay up late writing a post or reading reviews and commenting about your experience: Insomnia from running all that furious, righteous adrenaline through you all day.
7. Wake and immediately look for validation: Skip the morning workout or meditation and read what people said in response to your reviews.
8. Regret. Remorse. Repeat.

The feedback loop of crushing people online with data was toxic. Immediately after my searing posts went live, I would overeat. Then I would waste countless hours online, checking on how my reviews were doing. From there, I would stop listening to music I enjoyed, start to sleep poorly and, within 48 hours, I would start to be toxic to the people in my real life.

I had found the problem, but could I fix it? To remedy the situation, I made a conscious effort to leave more nice reviews, but the damage was done. Once I knew I had an audience, I became an actor, not a consumer; my feelings spread across the internet like contagions.

We owe it to each other to look very closely at the culture of mass shaming we find ourselves in now. Some things are better left unsaid.

Call it digital karma or the e-law of attraction; it doesn't matter—what matters is how we end up treating ourselves.

Whether we're avoiding a line at the local fast food restaurant with an app, finding the perfectly reviewed item or getting one last gotcha in while venting about a bad experience, what we put into the universe always comes back to haunt us.

Here are three ways I shaped my happiness by plugging into the opinion and customer feedback systems in positive ways. Don't unplug, connect differently.

OPINION TIPS

- ✦ **YOU NEED CASHIERS:** How dealing with people might save your sanity.

- ✦ **POPULARITY CAN'T BE TRUSTED:** Get more out of the internet by avoiding popular opinion.

- ✦ **NO MORE ANONYMOUS ASSHOLE REVIEWS:** Only leave good reviews for a week. You'll lose a few pounds and your sex life will get better.

YOU NEED CASHIERS
How dealing with people might save your sanity.

I'm not a coffee drinker, yet there is something exciting about the prospect of a large hot drink from a megacorporation. I don't know why, but I find it magical to have someone yell my name while holding a drink aloft that they've made just for me.

In 2015, Starbucks introduced mobile ordering. No cash, no having to say your order twice; waiting in line looking at your phone was a thing of the past. But waiting in line, paying for your drink and repeating yourself are, whether we admit it or not, important parts of life. Technology, for all the ways it creates more time for us, is slowly removing the most important parts of our interactions. There is inherent value in waiting, interacting with people and actually paying for things. Look around you right now. We have people do everything for us, and when we don't have these services, this endless access to convenience, we lose our minds. What kind of world have we created? If there is any sense of entitlement, I would argue it came from the App Store, not economic disparity.

As a 50-year-old gay Buddhist, I'd like to juxtapose two ideas about your opinions and your technology. First, the gay man in me wants you to think about the 1964 hit "People" by Barbra Streisand and its first line: "People who need people are the luckiest people in the world." Next, the Buddhist philosopher in me wants you to step back 20 years earlier to 1944 and consider French existentialist Jean-Paul Sartre: "Hell is other people."

These opposing ideas are the foundation of the most important relationship advice I can give you in this book. It's simple: don't avoid people.

We avoid people all the time with technology. Technology

is basically a queuing system for how much humanity we can handle at once. Consider a few ideas: Only give your feedback to someone who can do something about it. Don't fill out surveys or respond to survey calls, and at the very least, never, ever sign up for reward club cards.

This is important: complaining to technology about poor processes is no different from spitting into the wind—the wind doesn't care, and you end up covered in drool.

What I advocate is abandoning all the technology we use to avoid interacting with humans one day a week—by ordering food online, leaving anonymous feedback on a website or rating anything in an app. What you will slowly find out, after just two days of dealing with people, is that first, we are woefully underpaying people who deal with crap problems; and that second, people, almost all of them, are really, really just like you.

The person being skimpy with your toppings at Chipotle probably doesn't want to be there, and even a $15-per-hour nationwide minimum wage will not make their day all that much better. Yet, if you skip ordering ahead online, smile, ask them how they're doing and ask them questions about your order like it's your first time, well, that will do a few things: First, you'll get a lot of food, with toppings galore. Second, they will get to speak about the food they are preparing, which is something they are likely quite knowledgeable about. And finally, you will both feel a thousand times better than a Facebook like has ever made you feel.

This tiny tech hiatus will not be easy. When I stopped using automation in 2016 to focus on people one day a week, people thought I was out of my mind, or worse, judged me for not being as efficient as they were. True, you will run into cashiers who don't want your chitchat. Talking to people during retail transactions is akin to heresy in some establishments—you are wasting everyone's time. But I promise you that if you take the time to look up, thank someone or thoughtfully say why you are disappointed—or pleased!—your day will be better.

POPULARITY CAN'T BE TRUSTED
Get more out of the internet by avoiding popular opinion.

Online opinions today have become a brand's biggest fear and a consumer's weapon of choice when things go wrong. I know it's going to sound unwise, but we need to try to buck the system. The power of going against popular opinion will, I promise, help you start to create more time in your life. We miss a lot because it is not popular. Do you suffer from product or service FOMO or "Faux-MO"?

Faux-MO, as I define it, is the condition of letting the internet confiscate your free will by taking over all your decisions. You can diagnose yourself with faux-MO by answering a few simple questions.

1. Have you ever considered how many reviews something had before you looked at the price?
2. Do you Google for problems before you make a purchase?
3. When you look for a room on Airbnb, do you read the reviews first?

Instead of using the internet's ranking look at a brand's website—how do they handle support? Search Twitter for how a brand responds to people. Don't miss out on opportunities, products and experiences just because the internet hasn't ranked them yet.

NO MORE ANONYMOUS BAD REVIEWS

Only leave good reviews for a week. You'll lose a few pounds and your sex life will get better.

This last tip is one that will transform you in less than 24 hours. We have all been there, those days when we take our anger out on the first stranger we see. But I have found the key to happiness, reputation and influence in the world is this: be a nice person, on purpose, online, as if it was your job, for 24 hours. I mean, change someone's world with a review.

The exercise goes like this: Take three times in your day where something happened, good or bad, and write a review of the situation with the most positive feedback you can find. Go online and write the most amazing review about anything you can find that was positive about the experience. I promise that without fail you will sleep better that night. There is something truly transformative about the power of positivity in digital systems.

✧ ✧ ✧

Next stop on my digital lifestyle train: content and content creation. I was about to become part of the creative economy and gain control over my own destiny by applying the principles of attention, time and big data to guarantee myself a future in this complicated digital existence.

PART THREE

INFORMATION
(2010-2012)

Content, Work and Money

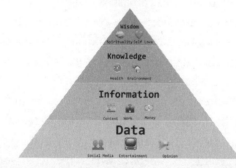

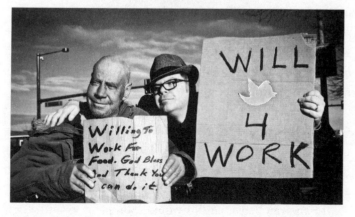

"It's not information overload. It's filter failure."

—Clay Shirky

The process of advancing your career outside of traditional roles was upended by the early part of 2010. Employees were gaining and maintaining high-traffic blogs, creating and producing valuable podcasts and even spending their own dollars to create a brand unto themselves.

Unless you're a tradesperson, you are likely succeeding or failing based solely on how you're using your tech. Let that sink in for a moment. No matter who you are, you are probably measured and evaluated on your successful use of technology.

Maybe it's the documents you create, the spreadsheets you crunch, the word count you amass, the number of retweets you get or the views on a video, but we are all measuring and being measured by someone, somewhere, somehow. So you can either be the person creating what gets measured or you can be the person deciding what gets measured.

We don't often talk about work this directly, but that's all there is to it. In this part of the book, I want to talk about why I chose to move to content creation and what that means. After that, we can get into the weeds of what it means to work. First, let's go make something of ourselves and our career.

I decided to add a new category of information alongside work, one I called "content creation." Building content for a business pays the bills today; saving that content online pays the bills tomorrow.

In a world of content creation, applications like email and Google Docs would for the first time really take center stage in the catalog of my life. My calendar, which had never really moved out of the spotlight since I was eight, would take on even more importance.

In an even bigger shift, I would soon pivot toward a new category of technology to contain my life library. In 2010, I started harnessing the power of document-sharing services: Pressfolio, Dropbox, SlideShare and SoundCloud are work services, not applications. They are platforms or sites that take the work product I make as a content provider and make them accessible to the world. They ultimately allowed me a new source of information with which to construct and understand my impact on the digital world.

The last area I would bring online was finances, or what I refer to in my data silo as money. In the wake of my early and prolific use of social media, I had finally managed to hold on to a stream of steady jobs with increasingly hefty paychecks. Now that I didn't have to live paycheck to paycheck, I wanted to see where my absolute lack of control when it came to money stemmed from. I needed to understand why and how I spent money, because it was the ultimate drug of choice for a consumption-aholic like me. And sure enough, the lessons I learned about how I spent money would shape and change me.

6

Content:
Will Work for Tweets

The Internet Is Your Brand and Identity

DIGITAL LEGACY

We live in a digital economy, which simply means most of what we consume is intangible—we can't hold it. More often than we care to admit, we are passively consuming this material. Not only do we *not* have a hands-on relationship with it, but we don't even realize we are consuming anything. There is no single greater reason to consider joining the ranks of the creative class.

There is no industry on Earth that is not being torn asunder by the conversion to digital content. Even electricians, plumbers and lawyers will soon be YouTubing their way to new customers. So let's sit around the kitchen table and have the uncomfortable talk about selling out to the internet. You have to start creating something. Maybe it's a Pinterest page with your favorite room designs, or maybe it's a clickbait blog on LinkedIn. Heck, live-streaming your daughter's dance recital counts, but what really matters is why you are doing it and what you will gain.

Let's start with what you will gain: you will gain nothing, for now anyway. But don't worry, that's the goal in the beginning. A body of work is just that: a mass of material for others to review or give up on. No matter if you're a family of four with your weekly vlog series on YouTube or you're about to set sail into retirement with your GoPro and a round-trip ticket to the world, it's time to build an online body of work.

The work serves as both a conversation starter and, more importantly, if you're still in the prime working part of your life, it's what future employers will review. It's ok to have a Facebook full of political rants as long as you have an impressive set of blogs too. Content for content's sake can feel cheap; that's not what I'm advocating. Just start thinking about how to slowly build a body of photos, videos or text that represents what you're good at.

BECOMING A MOUTHPIECE BY TYPING A LOT

My journey with content finally led me to a true understanding of *algorithmic influence*, or what marketers like to call *influence marketing*. In other words, big companies that no one trusted paid guys like me big money to tell other people they were good, responsible, benevolent behemoths. While this lined my pockets, ultimately, it also led me to a deeper understanding of the legacy I needed to leave online.

As a result of my relatively early pivot to social media for professional use back in 2008, I had somehow turned myself into a mouthpiece for the industry that, ironically, no longer had a job for me. Once I crossed that threshold from technical consultant to sales engineer, the dark path to marketing and PR wasn't far behind. Oh, that enchanted forest of industry conferences, full of male-dominated keynotes and well-meaning codes of conduct, a decade late and a few women short.

I made it to my fortieth birthday living life as a "computer person," as my mom would put it. My career path was pretty typical—a series of relatively standard-issue IT positions over a 20-year period of time, only hindered by my constant trips to HR. The software companies I worked for make solutions that are used by Fortune 500 companies around the world. The larger umbrella industry I was part of is referred to as *enterprise technology*, a really fancy way of saying the shitty software you have to use at work. These legacy enterprise technology companies—whose names read like a whatever-happened-to list at your high school reunion—include places like Oracle, Lotus, IBM, SAP, all of which were industry leaders in their day, playing important roles in the fusion that would unite work and the internet between 1998 and 2008.

After I was laid off from my job as a business development vice president at LANDesk in 2008, I became obsessed with how much my own industry was failing to keep up with consumer technologies. I got busy tweeting out sharp criticisms of organizations, companies and other industry peers. Twitter was and still is a microblog service—the perfect foundation for millions of people who would take to mobile lifestyles; as a content service, it was and is unstoppable. I was, for lack of a better term, a one-man Twitter ringmaster for the dying IT support industry.

Just think about how often you read something online and an old tweet is documented in the body of an article. Even the Library of Congress archived tweets from the president until, well, the president ate Twitter.

So my first real stop on the content wagon was building a following on Twitter. All my hustling and tweeting paid off, because in November 2010 I was "acqui-hired," a ridiculous term millennials and old-timers created in the tech media for hires when their startup was closing up shop and their brand was being absorbed into a bigger organization. I would be joining that IT training organization in Canada called Pink Elephant to help them get a handle on how to take advantage of the age of social media. Or something like that. What it really meant was that I could stop worrying about a paycheck and focus on being even more disruptive.

REEL VS. REAL TIME

Something else that intrigued me was happening around this time. The world's fascination with current events had evolved into the world's need to discuss and participate in trending events. (The first time I saw a tweet from CNN about Netflix being down, I knew we had entered a time where history was being written by the speed of our connections rather than the content of our lives.)

I had also begun hosting a weekly podcast. I recorded *ITSM Weekly* with two other high-profile social media content providers, Mat and Mat. The idea was simple: if I could capture the attention of the IT support industry, then I could continue to get asked to speak and expand my footprint as the go-to guy in the new social media age. It was time to start expanding my reach for the one thing I was well-known for: harnessing social media as a platform for career manipulation.

With a successful podcast (it was number one in the IT industry), a growing Twitter following and the backing of a global education company in IT like Pink Elephant, it was time for me to marry Silicon Valley to the old-school IT department help desk.

Fusing my career with the content I was creating online advanced my reputation, increased my salary and slowly expanded my viability in new industries. But I worried: Would all this content come back to haunt me?

The nuptials I wanted to encourage between IT support and Silicon Valley started the day I reached out to a small help desk software company called Zendesk. Zendesk was already a Silicon Valley darling and much ballyhooed in that middle world where customer support meets IT help desk. The company is led by an amazing Dane named Mikkel Svane. Mikkel, luckily enough, happened to like my style on Twitter and was a decent man, so I thought we could help each other out. Next, I contacted Hootsuite, the popular social media management platform. I knew their CEO, Ryan Holmes, had been aware of my usage and presence, so I asked Hootsuite if they wanted to sponsor a tour, along with Zendesk, for me to go to different chapters of the HDI, the Help Desk Institute. (Yes, you read that right. There is a membership organization to console you for working a help desk job.) The goal was to demonstrate to support professionals how to use social media not only for their own careers but as an IT tool.

I built a strong business case for why Hootsuite and Zendesk needed me to go out on a roadshow. In my opinion, the IT support industry was avoiding social media, and they hadn't yet woken up to the fact that Hootsuite, the tool to monitor feedback online, was the perfect way to help IT see its power. Furthermore, I knew that the new breed of IT support, such as Zendesk, needed to get a foot in the door of traditional old-stogie organizations that didn't trust cloud software.

I needed to convince everyone that paying me a mere $5,000 for this tour, plus covering all my travel expenses, was beneficial. (This, I will point out, was a lot of money for me at the time.) I would come armed with a mountain of metrics, like the number of page views the slides I was presenting had received, as well as videos of those presentations filled with bumpers (those advertisements that come before you watch a video), in order to show them the impact, financial and otherwise, social media could have on their businesses. My goal was to demonstrate to my sponsors that this roadshow would have a greater economic impact on their bottom line than any paid Google advertisement.

Sure enough, I had been right about the need for this kind of information. After the tour was over, the slides I had been using on the roadshow were racking up thousands of views on SlideShare and Vimeo. Both industries, IT support and Silicon Valley tech startups, took notice.

If I couldn't change the industry fast enough from the inside, I would have to go outside and knock on the front door. I needed to save my profession, even if that meant being forced out of my old career.

WATCHING YOU WATCHING ME

The entire time I was on the road showing my new topics to audiences, I kept noticing something else happening on SlideShare. People were stopping to view certain slides more than others. I could see how many people were clipping certain slides and saving a copy.

It turns out that people really liked it when I talked about the future and used screenshots of applications. More importantly, any slides that had numbers, projections or stats, some of which was pure speculation on my part, were instantly more popular with my audiences. This insight would be critical as I created new slides and presentations in the future. I was turning all my data into information.

I was now in a prominent position within this global community. My podcast for the industry, *ITSM Weekly*, was expanding with a UK edition, my slides on SlideShare had been shared over 50,000 times, my work Twitter following was close to 4,000, which was not bad in those days, and there wasn't a person in our industry who hadn't at least heard of me. I was thrilled to be honored by the itSMF, an older, yet still influential, community of IT practitioners, with their 2010 President's Award.

In less than two years, I went from being an undesirable, laid-off, LANDesk software VP to being an influential, award-winning industry icon, one tweet at a time, and with a show on iTunes to boot. *That* was the power of content and influence online at the dawn of the mobile age.

It doesn't matter what field of work you're in, you have to start to create a digital legacy. That means creating content on the web. Maybe it's Facebook posts, Tweets, blogs, podcasts, live-streaming your shopping sprees or Instagramming your latest dinner. Your work today and soon tomorrow will be partly evaluated on the following you have for the content you provide.

To that end, you need to think about three areas of your online life to bring meaning to the content you create: first, getting your content noticed; second, creating new content; and third, promoting what you do.

Create something, get noticed, learn something new and repeat—but whatever you do, don't unplug.

CONTENT TIPS

+ **THINK LIKE A MACHINE:** How to get noticed by thinking about how a machine sees your data.

+ **EDUCATION IN YOUR INBOX:** Use web alert tools to learn new things and stay current in your career.

+ **BUYING THE STAIRWAY TO HEAVEN:** Use old-fashioned connections and cash to get noticed.

THINK LIKE A MACHINE

How to get noticed by thinking about how a machine sees your data.

Creating content is easy enough now. Getting people to consume your content is the holy grail of the next decade.

As a word, "algorithm" is not new; it has centuries-old roots in the Greek word *arithmos*, meaning number, yet it hasn't been this casually tossed around since Plato ate grapes near a fountain in Athens.

Actually, algorithms are just pieces of software that move information around. Google has algorithms to make sure you see what you want to see every time you search, Facebook has them to make sure you see your aunt's pie first when you log in and YouTube has them to show you the latest woodworking video from your favorite hardwood artisan the moment you leave the trending section of the site.

Algorithms are written by people. (Well, at least for now. Discussing the machines that write their own software would be an entirely separate book.) Let's focus on where algorithms come from.

Think about Facebook. Facebook's goal is to keep you online wasting time for as long as possible. It's as ugly to type as it is to live, but that's the reality. If you wanted to keep someone someplace for a long time, you would first consider all the things they like, then you would make sure those things were easily accessible.

For better or worse, the world runs on code, and that means that millions of tiny decisions are made for you each and every day. In fact, the number of unseen factors in your life that decide your fate for you would probably scare you. This is your opportunity to dive in and participate in the matrix of code swarming around you.

You have crafted the perfect Facebook post, snapped the

most stunning photo or captured the coolest moment on video. Posting it and allowing others to enjoy it is easy, but you're now interested in getting noticed. What do you do? You think like an algorithm.

The first group of people who will see your post are the people who always comment on or like your creations. You know, that gaggle of old faithfuls who, within moments of a post, send you hearts, likes or quick memes.

These people are the easiest win. The programmer of your online world knows that if you post something, it should be shown to your old faithfuls first.

But how do you get your post noticed by more than just your regulars? You could have a popular friend reshare your content. Or you could constantly reshare it, maybe each day posting the same thing over and over. But people will likely continue to ignore you or start to actively dislike you.

Remember, we want you to get noticed by employers or people willing to pay you, in money or attention, for your creations. So look at the tools available to you when you post and think like an algorithm.

What is a Facebook post really? Well, it's the actual text you write or the photo you post, correct? Not really—that is the smallest part of a post. The machine doesn't read your words or see your photo, but the machine or algorithm does have hundreds of data points it looks at.

Let's deconstruct a post and look at it like a machine. Say I post a photo with a few choice sentences under it. This seems simple, but behind this post there are a ton of things going on.

The source of the photo: Was it a cell phone camera or something else? If it was a cell phone camera, was it taken with the front-facing camera or the back-facing camera? Is this photo from Friday at 11 p.m. or Monday at 1 p.m.? Now, is the photo raw, or did you change the photo with a filter or add words to it? Next, is this post out of character for you, do you normally even post photos? Did this post come from your phone or did you create it on your laptop? What about location, is this photo from someplace you traveled to away from home? When you posted the photo, did you check in to a location or add a feeling tag, like happy, excited or scared? Did you use words that were out of character or boring? Unfortunately, the list of characteristics in a Facebook post would fill the remaining pages of this book.

What could you do to fool the algorithm into ranking your post higher? You could post your content at a time you don't normally go online, or you could add a location and take time to say exactly how you're feeling. There is even software to schedule your posts so that they don't match what your friends and Facebook expect from you. It's the automation equivalent of robocalling for feedback.

The systems we use every day feed on data. If I want my friends to notice something, I add a location to the post and boom, I get two times more likes and comments. If I really need attention, I add one of Facebook's 51 emotions. (Isn't it ironic that they only offer five emotions to respond back to a post with?) Creating a post with a "feeling happy" literally rockets your content to the top of the feed for your friends. If you really want attention, ask your Facebook community to help you with a recommendation. Suddenly everyone you ever knew is chiming in with help.

Those days when you feel a bit low and wonder why your posts about life's ups and downs don't get the same support as the one where you're looking for a new dry cleaner, the answer is simple. The data from your post isn't as compelling to your friends' feeds, because the goal is to keep them logged in.

Advice about where to shop is infinitely more engaging than how you navigate depression.

This is it, the really scary truth of online friendships. Sadly enough, if you want to be connected to the world online, you have to think about the data of those connections, not the people behind the data.

EDUCATION IN YOUR INBOX
Use web alert tools to learn new things and stay current in your career.

Not a lot of my work hacks made it through the decade with me, but one did. It was my ability to stay on top of trends and make sense of all the news and new information in the world. That hack, we will call it the "stay-ahead-of-the-curve hack," uses a tool available to everyone called Google Alerts. My first Google Alert was like most of my social media career in the early part of the 2000s, a vanity play. Anytime "Chris Dancy" showed up on a website, I would get an email from the service to show me the page that had mentioned me.

But I knew I could use Google Alerts for something more than feeding my ego. I wanted Google to teach me something new, one email at time. Robotics, automation, biohacking, wearable technology or augmented reality, it didn't really matter. The world of technology was changing so quickly, that's how I needed to learn about it—in an endlessly updating stream of information.

I created conference presentations, complete with titles, topic descriptions and takeaways. I never let on about the one small important item missing from the equation: I had no idea what I was talking about.

There is a very long tail when it comes to innovation, which means you don't need a lot of history to be relevant, you need a lot of *recent* history. After constructing the topics for my talks each year, I would then set up Google Alerts that matched the talk titles. I set up my systems so that I was drip-fed information and innovation every day for nearly half a decade.

When I got an alert that tweaked my interest and matched an upcoming presentation, I would save the full article, references and photos in Evernote, the web-clipping tool used by millions. That service became the backbone of what would evolve into my real-time archive of technology's biggest trends. When it came time to give a new talk, I would simply open Evernote, copy the notes into a PowerPoint, and within a few hours, I had a fully formed presentation.

I continued to share these presentations on SlideShare and amassed thousands of views.

My ability to manage thousands of pieces of information in real time was helping advance my career and my industry, and soon enough, the rest of my life as well.

BUYING THE STAIRWAY TO HEAVEN
Use old-fashioned connections and cash to get noticed.

Hands down, the best way to create content and grow a following is to focus on what you are passionate about and let the world discover you. Unfortunately, there is so much to see in the digital wild that being found is akin to stumbling on Darwin's orchid. So be bold: ask an influencer or someone with more popularity for their help in getting you noticed. If you don't have the network or the courage to reach out to a famous stranger, then there is the second way: buy that access. Today, there are vending machines in Asia that sell Instagram likes, and you can find websites that will sell you an instant following on Twitter or more YouTube views than Justin Bieber. Unfortunately, these shallow attempts at instant credibility don't hold water in the long run, and it's easy to spot when you're faking it.

Most services where you want to be discovered, including Facebook, YouTube, Instagram and Twitter, have advertising arms for small businesses. Think of how many times you have seen "promoted" under a piece of content on your social sites. One of the interesting things about promoting content as a person and not a business is how strangely empowering it can be. Once I was in Australia at a conference and I took a photo of the beach and put it on Facebook. Later that day, Facebook suggested that I promote the image. I thought to myself, *Why in the world would I pay to promote a beach picture to my friends?*

But back in 2012, it was starting to become obvious as I researched content and work strategies that it would take more than sheer effort to get people to pay attention. I took a chance and spent $10 on the photo. Suddenly my beach photo was liked, commented on and shared all over my Facebook feed. Did I really just spend $10 to get my friends to notice my vacation? Yup, that's how social media works. It's the dark underbelly of social media that is greased with cash. But there's not much point in looking at this system with disdain; what I'm encouraging you to do is explore it.

Facebook will let you advertise any post or link to external content. You can narrow who sees it by selecting certain demographics, like geography or age. Don't want your friends to know you're pimping out your world-famous chocolate cake photos? Target your post to 60-year-old women in Eastern Europe. Done. Suddenly you have a following, although your fan club meetings are held in Budapest.

This targeting works on all social media platforms and is actually pretty easy. Maybe you're a mom, student or scared project manager in an IT department like I was. Create a piece of content, a blog, photo or video or even record yourself humming a song. Now head to Facebook, Google Ads or Twitter, search for "advertisement," and you're on your way.

For only $5, you can gain access to a bunch of new people who might enjoy your content, plus you'll start to understand the mechanics of online influence. Getting noticed in a world where no one has time for the most heartfelt post is hard, so maybe we need to think about greasing the emotional wheels a little. It's long been rumored that Taylor Swift's father had a hand in making sure she was the opening act for headliners in her early days. Maybe that football scholarship had more to do with a player's YouTube views for that Hail Mary pass than that player's football skills. Maybe the game is all around, all the time.

Did I buy my way to the top? Did I emotionally pimp myself to the front of the Facebook feed of my friends? Yes, there were times I did engage in all these behaviors to understand the mechanisms behind them. But for me, it was well worth it. There is no reason not to take to the internet with a vengeance about your content or your passions. Get noticed, get loud, do what it takes, take to the silicon streets. This is your chance.

What did I do with all this influence and my new career as a budding technologist and world-class speaker? I made sure that I climbed the corporate ladder while my star was shining. Or, as RuPaul says, "You better work."

7

Work:
Never Reply to All

People Work with Your Habits, Not You

HACKING WORK

In the first section of this book, I shared with you the invisible strings that tied me to social media and how I used those connections to come to terms with my behavior and understand how online tools could manipulate my friends and me. Today, Facebook and other large companies are facing charges of being careless with our data, manipulating our feelings and possibly helping to influence elections around the world.

I examined how simple everyday entertainment tools like Spotify, Apple Music or Pandora shaped my productivity and how Netflix aided and abetted me in binge-eating. Using the data about what I passively absorbed into my psyche, I came to realize how these tools were editing my hours and creating new habits. We have yet to see how destructive this constant distraction can be collectively. But just as smoking wasn't a problem until it was, sometime in the next few years the consequences of this abuse of our attention—using the internet as a constant distraction—will finally be exposed.

Finally, by examining how and when I used the internet to weaponize customer service, it became evident that I needed to be mindful of the value of my opinion online. The tools and constant requests to share my experiences had turned me into a real jerk when things didn't go my way. In so many ways, the power of one unhappy voice and a progressively faster echo chamber is now reshaping all of us.

The hundreds of connections I mapped, cataloged and reviewed between 2008 and 2010 were both enlightening and life-altering, shaping how I looked at every other part of my life.

WHITE-COLLAR COAL MINER TO MILLIONAIRE

Up until 2010, I had done what every single person of my generation with a white-collar job had done to succeed in their career: get a job, do it well, learn how to do something new and start over. From 1990 to 2010, as a help desk technician, software consultant and pre-sales engineer for enterprise IT systems around the United States, my career, while good, wasn't a remarkable Silicon Valley story of success.

In 1990, at the age of 24, I was making approximately $25,000 a year, and by the end of 2010, at 40 years old, I was bringing home close to $100,000 a year. Not a bad increase for a kid whose parents said during a family dinner in 1986, "Get an accounting degree, those computers will never take off."

My current journey started in 2008 with a small consulting firm I founded called ServiceSphere with the severance pay from my last job. While this wasn't always a lucrative time, consulting allowed me to study how work had changed between 2000 and 2010.

The consulting company, which gave rise to my podcast,

prolific tweet storms and delivering keynotes at small IT events around the United States, firmly established me in two ways. First, it helped me understand how content drove the metrics around online authority, influence and perceived importance. Yes, the content I created and put online from 2010 to 2012 not only defined who I was, but more importantly it signified how important I was, at least to the algorithms that measured connectedness.

Nothing could prepare me for the career ride between 2010 and 2015. In those five years, I would go from $100,000 a year to close to half a million a year. From local speaking events with 10 to 15 people huddled in a conference room to concert halls with 5,000 to 15,000 attendees hanging on my every word.

I've met with and consulted for major tech companies, from Google and Twitter to Microsoft and Salesforce, because I made calculated decisions about my career and my time. Sometimes these decisions were disastrous and other times they paid off.

I'm like you: I have good days and bad days at work. The only difference is, I measured every single one and learned what worked and what didn't in the age of always-on, open-office, coworking bliss.

ROCK SUPERSTAR

I was listening to Cypress Hill's "Rock Superstar" in my earbuds, working on a presentation for my talk at ServiceNow's annual user conference in 2011 in San Diego. My temporary career with Pink Elephant was in the rearview mirror, and I was out to make sure I impressed not only the attendees at the event but also the executive staff.

My online bantering with the heads of all the big software companies in the United States had landed me an invite to this upstart's annual cloud conference. Long before the cloud was everywhere and part of every product, companies like Salesforce and ServiceNow were pioneering work from a browser.

Now that I had their attention, I would blow them away at their conference and work my way to the front of the line at this company. I mean, I had what it took, a history in IT, an attitude for disruption and a vast online audience.

At that time, my 15,000 followers online were split between people who also followed ServiceNow and those who followed the number-one competitor in the IT business at that point, BMC. I was sitting squarely in the sights of the two most significant software companies in my industry.

The annual conference for ServiceNow came and went. Within a few weeks I received an email from their head of online community asking if I would like to join the company in an executive role. This was a major step forward for me; no longer was I just a washed-up fortysomething exec, I now had a job at the most innovative company in the industry.

I announced my partnership with ServiceNow on my blog, and my little IT community lost their minds. People thought I had sold out. How could I go to work for a *vendor*?

I did not plan to retire at ServiceNow. The job was a stepping-stone to creating more content and furthering my ambition of understanding cloud and mobile software. I would benefit from ServiceNow, and they would benefit from saying they employed me.

My rock-star status had been cemented. ServiceNow splashed banners across their landing page announcing my webinars and events.

Who among us hasn't wondered what they get paid to do? Do you get paid to send email, make your sales numbers, create PowerPoint presentations? Whatever you get paid to do, there is a way to measure it, and trust me, someone somewhere is doing just that. With my new job, I decided to start measuring how I worked.

During my time at ServiceNow, I collected all sorts of work statistics: when I sent an email, when I got an email, what hours I worked, when was I productive, who I met with, what I got done. I started measuring tasks: How often did I begin a new one, finish it, delay doing it? How and when did I procrastinate?

EMAIL KILLS CAREERS BUT SO DOES BEING ON GOOGLE

In my attempt to better understand how I spent my time at work, I decided to up my data game a bit. With a few simple codes, I automatically recorded when I received an email; what I did with that email after I received it; all documents created, modified and deleted and various other stats. Every time someone sent a reply all to say "Thanks" and cc'd 400 six-figure professionals, I added it to my personal database. Within weeks, I had tens of thousands of data points showing how much I was working for ServiceNow.

Data entries from work were color-coded in shades of red. Email was blood red, and soon my calendar was covered in this deep red from each email arriving in my inbox, sometimes several per minute.

By understanding how I worked, I could start to focus on specific tasks at certain times. I needed to get the big stuff, the creative stuff, out of the way in the morning before I looked at my inbox or I would get sucked into answering emails for hours.

✦ ✦ ✦

As had happened before in my career, my time at ServiceNow would be cut short because of my inability to play well with others. While the founder, Fred Luddy—a true visionary and

someone I consider to be a mentor more than an executive—
loved the way I worked, I was perceived as a threat to many
people I met.

If you were in marketing, you disliked me because I got
away with murder online. I could tweet, post and say what I
wanted with impunity. If you were in sales, you disliked me
because potential customers often only wanted to hear from
me because they followed me online. Legal and HR obviously
always had their hands full negotiating the weekly reports
about how I was out of control or less than professional.

My career ended when a member of the new executive
team reported that I was rude to a part-time marketing person.
How was I rude you might ask? During our initial meeting
when asked what I did for ServiceNow, I laughed and said,
"Just Google me." Apparently, the flippant attitude didn't go
very far in winning friends and influencing people.

Within a few weeks, I was in HR and being told that I
wasn't any more important than anyone else at work, regardless of how "Googleable" I was. The founder and the new executive team fought over my role. The writing was on the wall, but
something more profound was happening as half the team
fought to save me and half the team wanted me out.

MARKETING DEPARTMENT OF ONE TO MANY

A new style of employee had been hatched. One whose online
reach far exceeded their real-world worth. It was a sign of the
times for 2012. I was Trumping long before it was presidential
and I was suffering the backlash.

The lessons from this time in my career are important. No
matter how influential you become at your office or in your virtual world, one rule holds true: don't let your online shadow
cover up your real-world worth.

My online audience was huge, but I relied too much on

who I was online and forgot that people in the real world didn't care who I was in the virtual world. Unlike Wade from *Ready Player One*, the Ernest Cline nostalgia bestseller about a young man who becomes famous in a virtual reality, my reality wasn't ready to be all online or connected.

✦ ✦ ✦

If my social media use got me hired at Pink Elephant in 2010 and my podcast made me a must-have asset for cloud upstart ServiceNow in 2011, my prolific online stature would herald the last move in my career within the IT industry.

By the start of 2012, I had nearly 18,000 Twitter followers, which at the time was huge and practically unheard of for an IT guy. I had thousands of LinkedIn connections, and I had spoken at IT conferences in Europe, North and South America, Asia and Oceania. I had created content on everything from managing a help desk to hiring and promoting robots in the workplace.

"Visionary," "futurist," "thought leader" were all labels given to me when introducing me to new people. The entire IT industry was on Twitter by 2012, and I was their leader, each tweet, podcast rant and keynote further cementing my place as the king of white-collar IT work.

After my time at ServiceNow, I moved to the number-one IT software vendor in the world, BMC Software. BMC had spent the last 20 years securing, acquiring and installing IT systems around the world for Fortune 500s. They were as common as IBM but less well-known to the general public.

However, BMC was aging and, like most of the Fortune 500s, was now considered legacy. Legacy is a nice way of saying, "We have to replace this piece of software soon." Legacy is the death adjective for software. I knew a thing or two about legacy. My career until the age of 40 was officially legacy and I had successfully rebooted it. BMC wanted me to help create and patent a piece of technology that would steal the crown back from younger, sexier ServiceNow.

BMC would foster two different events beyond the creation of this cool piece of technology. First, my career in IT would be superseded by the global media attention that would anoint me the world's most connected man. Second, I'd have to use my data to save my job.

First though, I would have to come out of my data closet.

✧ ✧ ✧

A piece of advice about your career: start going to conferences that have nothing to do with your industry. I faithfully attend two big conferences, Theorizing the Web and CyborgCamp. These IRL tribes have become an adopted family for my career. Theorizing the Web is an academic, think tank–style conference; I am basically the only non-PhD there. Meanwhile, at CyborgCamp, where emergent technologies meet real-world problems, I am pretty much the only person over 35.

CYBORGCAMP

In fall 2012, I was walking down a street in forever-hazy Portland, the early morning light on my face, and the city's food trucks starting to power up. I was on my way to CyborgCamp to meet Amber Case. Amber had been the keynote speaker for South by Southwest earlier that year. She mesmerized me.

My goal for CyborgCamp was simple: I wanted to meet other people who were doing edgy and new things with technology to examine their lives, and I wanted to compare notes. I wasn't a speaker, nor had I been invited. I had simply signed up as a civilian and paid to be there.

In black Sharpie, I had scribbled "H+" (biohacker shorthand for human plus, somewhere between a biohacker and a robot) and "QS" (quantified self) as my interests on my name badge. In a strange twist of fate, I decided to use my private Twitter handle instead of my professional one.

Amber Case came bounding down the steps and into the large conference room: "Helloo!" Her welcomes are always cartoonish, part yell, part yodel. I couldn't believe she was right in front of me. She started to live-stream with her cofounder, Aaron Parecki.

The morning's topics ranged from bitcoin to low-friction data collecting. A guy named Mike Merrill, who was publicly trading his life via a personal stock exchange, spoke. His life story would be sold to Jason Bateman in a few years, but for now, he was still just a local web celebrity.

I was in a room with cyborgs, bitcoin tycoons and a person selling his privacy. The saying goes: if you're the smartest person in the room, you're in the wrong room. I was in the right room. During the final morning break, when I had a moment alone with Amber, I took a deep breath and opened up my laptop to share my data-tracking project with her. Her eyes opened wide as I showed her each day of my Google calendar, filled with data points delineating everything I did, logged and felt.

"Oh *my God*, you have to share this with the people here, Chris. You must!" Amber's voice crackled with excitement. She has a way of making you believe in yourself and the world; it is both childlike and utterly inspirational. I shook my head, horrified. Amber took me by the hand and led me up to the breakout session board.

"Put your name up here. Now," she demanded.

The afternoon at CyborgCamp was to be filled with unconferenced sessions, which simply means there was no structure. You could sign up for a slot if you had a topic you thought should be discussed, and people attended whichever meetings they found most interesting.

With a sense of anticipation, alongside utter fear, I grabbed a blue whiteboard marker and filled my name in for a 1:30-to-2:15 p.m. time slot in the large conference room named Picard. Under my name, I scratched the words, "Digital Quantified Self, knowledge locker, @servicesphere @chrisdancy," adding my work Twitter handle so people could see that I had actual followers.

As one o'clock got closer and closer, the conference room started to fill up with freaks, geeks and other techy folks as word spread about what I was about to share. After a shaky introduction of myself and my four-year project, I opened up my slides. I started talking about how I was using Zapier, IFTTT and Yahoo! Pipes to move data from my phone, sensors, home and car to my Google calendar.

To my surprise, the room got quieter and quieter, as everyone there seemed to lean in and listen. I lifted up my shirt to expose the chest strap that was collecting my heart rate and the waist strap that was monitoring my posture. I revealed my BodyMedia band on my bicep, my NikeFuel band on my wrist, as well as the other sensors all over my body. Then I started sharing what my phone was doing.

"This app collects the background noise in a room. I log my feelings on this app. This one keeps track of the types of places I go and how I get there." With each revelation, the room became more and more interested. I felt like a stripper of sorts: with each metaphorical layer removed, I was revealing more and more of my cybernetic infrastructure until the room was virtually undulating in a data climax.

After about 15 minutes of nonstop talking, I finally paused. There were people all over the audience waving their hands. I tried to answer their questions as quickly as I could. All the while, I could see Amber out of the corner of my eye, sitting in the back of the room with a Cheshire cat grin on her face.

After my presentation, a man from the audience approached me.

"Hey, I'm Klint. I'm from *Wired* magazine, and I'd love to learn more about what you're doing."

YOU'RE TRENDING, NOW WHAT?

On February 22, 2013, I woke up around 9:20 a.m., ate a bagel and drank six ounces of orange juice. After breakfast, I checked my phone. In my inbox, there was a message from Twitter saying I had been mentioned online. Then another email came in. Then the tweet notifications started popping up. Within a few minutes, I had 20 alerts saying I was being mentioned online. I logged in to Twitter and my heart jumped out of my chest when I checked my notifications. The *Wired* article had gone up.

QUANTIFIED MAN: HOW AN OBSOLETE TECH GUY REBUILT HIMSELF FOR THE FUTURE, the headline proclaimed. Hovering just below the headline, there was a provocative photo of me I had taken the previous year. I was standing next to a homeless person who had been holding a sign that read, "Will Work for Food." Mine said, "Will Tweet for Work."

From the winter of 2013 to 2014, I was on the cover of *BusinessWeek*, interviewed live on Fox Business, heard all over the world on the BBC World Service and had a TED Talk under my belt. To this day, when people ask me, "Do you have a Ted Talk?" I reply, "Yeah, I have a TED Talk, but there are also three TED Talks about me."

CyborgCamp had put me squarely in the crosshairs of the global media and contributed to the fact that today you can go to Google and type "most connected," and I come right up. You don't have to type my name. You don't have to type "most connected man in the world," you can just type those two words.

✦ ✦ ✦

Back at BMC, luckily, the PR team had been on top of the story this time, so I wasn't blamed for blindsiding them. They knew I had talked to *Wired*, and lo and behold, they were planning a media circus. At this point, I was feeling a little more confident about appearing on TV. With a little added data vigilance, but nothing like what was to come in terms of my own health-hacking, I had dropped down to around 250 pounds, almost 50 pounds lighter than my all-time high. Not only could I talk about the weight I had lost, but more importantly, I wanted to focus on how none of us were using all this technology in service of ourselves. From the abuse of email marketing in the corporate world to the harvesting of our digital organs by Facebook and Twitter, in my opinion, there was nothing good coming for white-collar America. To me, that was the real story.

HUMAN RESOURCES, MEET MY DATA

One day that spring, I was sitting in a cramped office in the financial district of Manhattan with a media coach, prepping for yet another interview. My nerves were frayed. I was doing interview after interview, and the PR people from BMC were putting a lot of pressure on me to stay on message and get the corporate pitch into the answer for every question I was asked. My PR liaison, Jenny, was watching everything I said and did and sending her feedback to the home office. After about two hours of being recorded live for a mock *Good Morning America* segment, the media coach asked me to stay on message for the hundredth time and I lost it.

I stood up and stormed out of the room, swearing. I was not now, nor had I ever been, someone who was good at staying on script. Jenny followed me out to the hall to check to see if I was ok, and I'm ashamed to say I just let her have it. I was fed up with having a PR flunky putting words in my mouth, and I'm sure she was just as sick of babysitting a loudmouth employee hell-bent on saying whatever he wanted.

On the ride back to the Waldorf Astoria, I apologized for my blowup, but I also defended my actions and words. Once we were back at the hotel, I went to my room and called our CTO to tell him about my blowup. "Just shake it off, Chris. You're in the middle of some tough stuff, but you'll be fine."

That night, I asked Jenny to meet me for dinner and I decided to take some notes throughout, in case I needed to protect myself in the coming days and weeks. Over dinner, Jenny drank a little too much and started sharing her own challenges with her child and her new husband's ex-spouse. I felt bad for her, but I tried to keep the dinner mostly professional.

We met the next morning in the lobby of the Waldorf near the famous clock, but instead of heading to our next appointment, she immediately told me to call her boss. She had recommended that we cancel the rest of the press tour. I was told to fly back for a conference, then report to HR directly afterward.

I was devastated. Unemployment loomed yet again. I reached into the only bag of tricks that had worked for me this far, data. Looking back over the past week with Jenny, I started mining. I needed to find a pattern to show how much pressure I was under and furthermore, prove that Jenny was the cause of my breakdown. I went back and grabbed all the data I needed: our schedule, our cab trips, our vocal levels, our meals logged, the number of alcoholic drinks consumed, the emails sent, phone calls made, text messages screenshotted.

I created an entirely fact-driven narrative of the past week of my life. Then I submitted it to my boss, Bill, Jenny's boss and HR.

Over the next few weeks, an internal investigation would put me on alert about my outbursts, but Jenny would also get a dose of her own medicine. I had given HR and her boss mountains of evidence pointing to her own hostility toward me.

She might have felt threatened during my media interview, but I had every heartbeat, shallow breath and sleepless night captured that resulted from her behavior toward me. (HR looks very different in a future where not only are "these calls monitored for your satisfaction," but the biological signatures of anger, aggression and frustration are recorded and reviewed along with them.)

GOODBYE HELP DESK INDUSTRY

Shaken, I knew my time in this role was nearing an end. One last keynote for my friends in the IT industry. Next up, Birmingham, England, for a conference I had helped put together called Tomorrow's IT Service Future Today, TFT13.

On the morning of June 18, 2013, I sent a tweet, along with a link to my presentation. "You've seen the data, now move the needle, the future of the future. Quantified existence. #Tft13 #Sdi13." I raced down to the stage where I was due to present in about two hours. My Fitbit showed no sleep and my diet was nonexistent, yet I was energetic, filled with the motivation to do something, to make an impact. I was confident about my presentation.

Yet I knew the thing that would change the event was the running live view of my sensors. All of my devices were hooked up to show the data they were collecting in real time. I ran around checking all the connections. Fitbit, check. Wahoo TICKR, check. LUMO Lift, check. All my data was streaming to the massive screens overhead. I could feel my chest tightening with anxiety.

"I've done something unique this year," I started tentatively. I went on to explain how, next to my presentation on the jumbo screens behind me, the audience would be able to see a monitor that would, from time to time, flash with my biological data. My walking gait, my heart rate and my voice level were all being streamed real time to the monitors and live to the internet.

"As you can see I'm a little excited right now. Throughout the presentation, we can get [that number] down, or we can get it up and we can have a medical emergency."

The sweat was starting to stream off my head. I was feeling vulnerable, in a big way. But the audience laughed as I walked back to the podium, which relaxed me. Over the next 40 minutes, I waxed about being connected and the future of work. As I made awkward jokes about my life and lifestyle, you could have heard a pin drop.

People enjoyed my talk, but what they loved was actually watching my body's reaction to my talk. It was a biological theater of sorts; instead of a seventeenth-century operating room, this one worked in concert with the theater of the mind.

I had technology strapped to my body with systems reading my actions and automating my life every second of every day. I wasn't working with technology anymore; I was technology.

I would leave BMC soon, secure in how my data could save my job and mesmerize an audience. I would head into the deepest darkest parts of my life in order to uncover and examine my health, environment, mind and love.

Not a lot of people will become viral sensations or get hired from their podcast or YouTube channels like I did.

Work today is dependent on the content you create—see

the last chapter and think about how you interact with your employer.

There are three things I think every office worker needs to consider immediately if they want to continue to be viable within their industry: how they use email; what tools they use at work; and if they're selling out their online identity.

Yes, it's a rat race, but this is no time to unplug the rodents.

WORK TIPS

✦ **YOU GET THE EMAIL YOU SEND:** Send only the number of emails you want to receive yourself.

✦ **YOUR JOB, YOUR TOOLS:** Use tools that help you understand how you work.

✦ **DON'T WEAR A DIGITAL SANDWICH BOARD:** Don't become a social media shill for your company, unless you're in marketing.

YOU GET THE EMAIL YOU SEND

Send only the number of emails you want to receive yourself.

Email is the original digital technology we never took the time to talk about. I'm a monster about using email effectively, and the reasons are simple. Email is soul crushing, abusive, passive-aggressive and yet somehow still a system of record for countless HR investigations and courtroom litigation.

How can something so banal yet so critically important live in the same digital spectrum? For me, the secret to email came from a data hack I implemented back in 2010. My email data was really simple: as you know, each email I received and sent created an entry in my calendar. Instantly I could see days where I was just processing email versus time when I was actually getting stuff done.

Yet the secret to email came in a way I never expected.

While calculating the amount of time I was spending on email, I realized I was receiving almost exactly as many emails as I sent. Seems obvious, right? But it's not. The requests coming directly to you rarely, if ever, exceed the number of emails you are sending out. It's just like holiday greeting cards—if you stop sending them, you stop receiving so many.

So if you're drowning in email, send less email. The real magic to email is responding quickly or not at all. If you never reply to anyone, your email volume will go down drastically. Or if that won't work for you, try responding instantly instead. When you respond to email quickly, you train people not to message you unless they want to have the metaphorical ball back in their court almost instantaneously. No one wants that. Simply put, you can reply so fast that people learn it's the least effective way to communicate with you. Data shows that the people you respond to the fastest probably email you the least. Look for alternative ways to document communications with your team to avoid email when you can.

The challenge is finding a way to get and receive tasks and clarification of those tasks that live outside of a typical email timeline.

Email worked because it was tied to a single day that we all shared at one company or industry.

Now that much of the world, or at least the news cycle, is independent of your working day we need new communication tools.

Find tools that let you multitask with assignments from many different departments, organizations and collaborators. Today we have personal communication tools like Slack, Trello or even Apple Business and personal chat that can help you accomplish these goals.

YOUR JOB, YOUR TOOLS

Use tools that help you understand how you work.

In most offices, small businesses and professional organizations, there are a set of standard tools we are expected to use. More often than I care to admit, these tools are inclusive to Microsoft Office and a standard-issue Dell laptop. In the past decade though, we have seen the emergence of a new trend in corporate offices called BYOD, or bring your own device, the idea being that employees can be responsible for their own equipment. The smartphone was really the driving force behind the hardware shackles being lifted off our white-collar bondage.

Yet no matter how many trends come and go in technology, if you have a boss, you still usually have to work with their processes and tools. Many of the headaches we experience at the office are related to bad processes and subpar tools, which work in tandem to create the most miserable environment for getting a project done.

If you pull the covers back at many upstart incubators and startups, you'll find that not only do they allow device freedom, but they encourage you to have tool freedom as well. Use any software you want to get the job done. Need to find out what your clients think of an experience? Maybe you should sign up for a SurveyMonkey account, a popular web-based tool for collecting feedback from just about anyone for any reason. Ever wonder how some people seem to get more meetings crammed in while they travel than you do? Look into a subscription to TripIt Pro, the travel assistant for your smartphone that watches your inbox and creates itineraries for you on the fly.

I'm not here to teach you productivity enhancements—there are books and web gurus galore who can do a better job on that. Instead I'm here to suggest that you, where appropriate, abandon the tools and processes that are slowing you down. I advocate this knowing full well that the ramifications for some jobs could be disastrous. No nurse should use 23andMe to diagnose a patient. No lawyer should create LegalZoom living wills. And I shudder to think about a schoolteacher downloading lesson plans from a shared site. (Mind you, I have run into all three of these things—there is no shortage of people outsourcing their own jobs—but more on that later.)

I'm simply encouraging you to look at your job as you would your health, social media, finances or travel and see if there are tools to help make it easier for you to manage it.

Another benefit of choosing your own tools is creating workflows that help streamline your job. There are many services, like IFTTT or Zapier, that let you connect apps together to create complex mini-jobs inside of other apps. Say you need to send a thank-you email after a meeting. Connecting your email to your reminders and creating a rule to schedule an email after each meeting is very easy. We live in an age where management expects this type of independent thought, and I promise that the lessons you learn from finding your own tools will only help you, especially as uncertainty continues to grow around us all.

DON'T WEAR A DIGITAL SANDWICH BOARD

Don't become a social media shill for your company, unless you're in marketing.

Over the past decade, I have seen employers move from having marketing teams to asking entire departments to do their own marketing outreach. All you have to do is log in to LinkedIn, and you can see regular folks like you and I, with their digital sandwich boards strapped to their profiles, sharing the latest webinar or blog post from their boss or cozying up to their next employer by commenting on their less-than-witty white-collar memes.

So I want to be upfront with you as we look at our careers and the future. Do not, under any circumstances, become a mouthpiece for your employer unless your job is in marketing, and then only do it if you are paid for it. The cringeworthy posts by the office secretary on professional networking sites slowly turning into a clickbait machine should terrify you. LinkedIn has become a digital marketplace of 1980s flying eagle motivational posters. Let that be a warning.

Employers today are paying for your time at the office, but they are also using you to extend their brand. This is a slippery slope in my opinion. If your career becomes a brand machine for your employer and not for you, then new employers will see you as a cheap sellout and just another number for their head count of likes and follows.

Your current employer needs your online authenticity like a vampire needs to sleep in a coffin. Don't give it to them. If your employer asks you to share their latest blog or video or start following your boss, start looking for another job immediately. Seriously, you can do a lot of damage to your online reputation. The algorithms behind sites like Twitter, LinkedIn and Google can't be undone. When you spend all your time creating and shaping your employer's junk content, you ruin any chance you have of branding yourself.

This sounds pretty dramatic, I know, but listen closely. I used to tell my employers, "I'll lend you my name, but you'll give me your power and cash if I do." Think about it: Who do you trust most for their opinion of Tesla? Elon Musk, a factory worker at the car assembly plant in Freemont, California, or the marketing manager at Tesla? For me, I follow two people: the factory worker and Musk. Everyone between those two people is covered in corporate sludge.

Don't sell out to your employer, don't be an unpaid extension of their marketing arm unless you're in marketing and try to avoid connecting, linking, friending or following anyone you work with. The systems that count those connections aren't revealing the damage they are doing to your future prospects of getting recruited.

8

Money:
A Fool and His Apple Pay
Soon Part

You Can't Subscribe to Values

MONEY FOR NOTHING AND YOUR BITS FOR FREE

At the McDonald's outside of Nashville, Tennessee, the front door is covered in decals: Apple Pay, Android Pay, Uber Eats, Mastercard, Visa. Today, there are more combinations for how to pay for and receive your Big Mac and fries than there were items on the original McDonald's menu.

Money is one of the oldest systems we have at our disposal, and it's probably the first tool we learn about that has an effect on our lives. It can ruin relationships or save people from ruin. Yet money itself is just like the internet. It is invisible for the most part, it acts like a login and password to the things we need and it's never as fast as we want. Measuring money is often left to overly simple checkbook balances or complex retirement portfolio strategies. Money itself is more complex than simply saving for today; it is tied up in virtually all of the invisible connections of our digital lives.

Between 2012 and 2015, I spent between $20,000 and $30,000 a year to fund the hundreds of services, apps, hardware and devices I was using to track myself. I mention this because I didn't physically handle much of that money, nor could I actually touch most of the services and items I was purchasing. Have you ever looked at how much of your budget is tied to invisible items such as subscriptions to tech services like Spotify, Apple Music, Netflix or Amazon Prime? Is Netflix worth $10.99 a month if you only watch one movie? Is your iCloud subscription backing up your family photos worth it if you are only using 15 percent of your storage capacity? What is too little space? What is too much?

Some invisible purchases seem easy to justify. On the surface, Uber or Lyft, both popular ride-sharing services, seem legit (nefarious corporate politics and urban congestion aside). But upon further examination, by removing the payment process in securing a ride, what Uber and Lyft have done is conceal your usage, and concealing your usage is the oldest trick in the book for emptying your bank account.

Why is it that Spotify sends you an overview of what you listened to each year, Facebook gives you highlights of your annual photos and Amazon remembers the last time you purchased shampoo, but Uber and Lyft don't share how often you ride, how much you spent or what those precious feedback ratings are worth? It's simple: they don't want you to know what you're worth. If you saw how much you spent on taxis in 2017, because you were feeling lazy, you were running late or it was just too cold outside, you'd probably be horrified.

The next thing to do when looking at your digital life through the lens of money is to examine the nature of convenience. In other words, start thinking about what data you are sacrificing for the right to make sure you don't have to wait one second longer for anything. Ordering food to pick up or be delivered via an app is basically opting into a level of financial surveillance that we can't yet appreciate.

It really started back in 2004 when Steve Jobs bragged on-stage that iTunes had millions of users' credit card numbers saved, essentially creating a marketplace where users didn't have to pull out a form of payment, they could just click and buy. Soon enough, the App Store on your mobile phone became a vacuum for cash.

Amazon, probably the stealthiest tech predator on the planet, has patented a process to store your credit card information and home address so that you only have to click a single button to have virtually anything you want sent to you. Think about that: they have an actual patent—the thing that protects the invention of the light bulb and the development of lifesaving drugs. They got a patent to help facilitate your ability to give them private information about you, your family and your finances. In return, you have the privilege of forgetting just how much money you spend with them.

Then they go a step further and ask you for $119 a year so you can get Prime shipping. In other words, you are forking over more privacy and more data, not to mention more money, for the privilege of wasting less time waiting. If you have the "Amazon Prime Now" option, you can pay another invisible premium to have things sent to you in one hour or you can pick up your items at an Amazon Locker, available at gas stations all over the United States, within moments of ordering.

At this point, I thought I had my online life under control. What could possibly go wrong in a world full of invisible connections that I was just starting to navigate and unravel? The convenience of cash in a cashless society has to be analyzed

with great care to understand all the connections that are sucking your life dry. My tips for navigating financial life today hopefully will bring you some welcome relief.

MAD MONEY, OR HOW I LEARNED TO LOG MY FEELINGS THROUGH MY SPENDING

In my financial life, I knew that my overwhelming need to give gifts and emotional spending were as predictable as the sunrise. My friends, as well as my analog life coach, would often tell me that I didn't need to buy my friends. But promoting content to Facebook fans and Twitter followers is essentially the equivalent of buying a support network. Paying, in one way or another, for people to like you was by no means a new concept.

Late in 2012, I started tagging my mood when I spent money on pretty much anything. Lunch was tagged as a "meal" in Mint, my budget and finance app, but now it also received a tag of "tired" or maybe even "lonely." I used the old standby acronym I learned on one of my many trips to AA in the 1990s and 2000s: HALT—Hungry, Angry, Lonely, Tired. I started to log, throughout the day and night, if I was hungry, angry, lonely or tired. When any of those emotions popped up, I noted the behavior that followed.

What I noticed first was that I tended to buy people gifts after I had logged a high number of angry tags. If I spent a lot of time angry, I splurged on presents.

Likewise, I found that if I spent a lot of time logging lonely feelings, soon enough, there was a substantial hike in my food intake. As loneliness went up, so did calories, and I mean really, really bad calories. When the number of tireds started stacking up in my emotion logs, so too did the number of unnecessary purchases for myself. The sinister sister to emotional eating, for me, was emotional spending. Retail therapy was a crystal-clear sign I wasn't getting enough rest.

Hunger was a strange thing for me. As an obese human for my entire life, I really was either in one of two states: painfully overfed or on the verge of a nervous collapse from blood sugar drops. Financial health, like nutrition, can't be at the far reaches of either end of the scale. When I was hungry, it triggered two of my bad behaviors. First, I would often overspend by aggressively, relentlessly shopping. Second, I would purchase things I didn't really need.

Food shopping in particular, i.e., grocery store visits, correlated my hunger and spending issues with yet another bad behavior of mine. You know how when you go to the grocery store hungry, you always regret it?

Not only was I frequently going to the grocery store so hungry I couldn't think straight, I was also rewarding myself for accomplishing an annoying task by eating the wrong things. There's probably a reason the warm, freshly baked pizza display at Whole Foods is positioned at the end of the shopping experience, where you are far more likely to reward yourself for all the good choices you've made in the vegetable aisle with a low-nutrition, high-regret finale for your shopping spree.

The correlation between my finances and my nutrition was astounding. When I ate whole, healthy foods with the right balance of fats and proteins, I spent less money, on everything. If I had a little bit to eat before hitting Amazon, I spent less.

I was starting to see a pattern. But I still needed more data to understand what was going on with my wallet.

WHERE DID YOU SPEND ALL THAT MONEY? OR THE POWER OF SEEING LOCATION AND MONEY ON A MAP

My next life hack in the financial category would be related to location. In 2012, there was a new banking startup called Simple. Simple had a very basic online interface and an easy-to-use app. Simple allowed you to tag purchases, but it also allowed you to take photos of your receipts, the purchased items and so on. But what Simple did better than anything else at the time was geotag your transactions. If you went to the subway and bought a train pass, boom, your credit card swipe was tagged with the location of that subway. The power of seeing my spending marked on a map, alongside my mood while spending, was astonishing.

You don't need to be Nate Silver to see obvious correlations. Perhaps it's not surprising that you spend more money on eating out when you're out of town traveling for work. Pretty obvious, right? But as we move into a world where Airbnb becomes the default for where you stay when you're traveling, this conclusion has a substantial impact. Now when you're traveling, you have an option for a full kitchen to prepare meals. The financial impact of small changes like this were significant for someone who travels constantly like I do.

I wanted to see what else I could learn about my behavior based on locational spending. Getting a handle on my bar behavior was the first order of business.

Heavy drinking had to go if there was going to be any peace in my late 40s and beyond. If only there was a way to have someone or something tell me to stop after I had purchased my second pitcher of beer. What if I could get my bank to cut my credit card off? Think about the power of getting a message reminding you of the right thing to do when you're engaging in certain bad behaviors at a specific location, as a warning, as support. I decided to investigate what I could do with a geofence and my personal data. Geofences operate much like an invisible dog fence. That wire is buried under the yard, sending a signal to the dog's collar. It trains the dog not to leave the yard by shocking it if it gets near the fence. It's a little sad to watch something free, fluffy and four-legged stop on a dime, but it does remind us of the profound power of location data.

Geofences are only possible with smartphones. Actually, it's one of only a handful of sensors that made our original smartphones *smart* back in the early part of this decade. A GPS sensor allows your phone to know where you are. But this simple information is surprisingly powerful. These days, this information is used by your phone to suggest that you need to leave soon for an appointment or offers you a faster traffic-free route to your destination. This location information allows your phone to participate in and create a geofence, or an invisible outline around an area that your phone is aware of. Geofences provide situational context, and contextual information is what is driving our technology economy.

Contextual information is rooted in the idea that we could better help ourselves if only we were given access to information "just in time." For example, it really is no good to get restaurant recommendations for Austin, Texas, while you are vacationing in Paris. The problem with these systems is that context relies on information; and this information comes at a cost—the utter collapse of what we call privacy.

THE NIGHT MY IPHONE BECAME MY AA SPONSOR

For me, I saw geofencing as a way to curb bad behaviors in specific locations. For example, what if I could shut off all my spending at bars after 10 p.m.? What if I could get reminders to stay on budget when I was at the mall?

During the last days of my drinking career, going to the

Atrium, my favorite bar on South Broadway in Denver, was always a double-edged sword. Yes, seeing my drug dealer behind the counter made me feel welcome, but the impending hangover, let alone the days of panic attacks afterward, definitely dragged down my love for the place. About an hour into one of my last trips, after I had paid for my second pitcher of beer, my phone made an alert sound.

"Oh sweetie, you're in trouble with Doug!" the barmaid said, with a look of disapproval. It was common for Doug to start texting me to come home within an hour of my arrival, as he was well aware of what might happen if I didn't. But when I looked down at my screen, I saw that the message was from myself: "You're going to be tired and have a panic attack tomorrow if you don't leave now."

The barmaid leaned over and looked. "What is that?"

Much to my surprise, one of my little hacks was working. My credit card knew I was at the bar, it was after 10 p.m. and I had already bought two pitchers of beer. Here was my trigger to get out of the bar immediately.

Seeing a note I had sent to myself in the future, the future that was happening right here, right now, was too much for me. I left the pitcher on the table and headed back home. That night, big mother, not big brother, arrived in the form of my iPhone.

HEY, BIG SPENDER: HOW I GOT CONTROL OF MY RUNAWAY SHOPPING WITH GOOGLE GLASS

My cyborg friend Amber Case soon helped me with my next financial hack when she came for a visit. After CyborgCamp, Amber and I had started talking a lot; she inspired my quest to think about who I was and what I was becoming, all wired up and driven by data.

Amber and her cofounder Aaron Parecki were the Sonny and Cher of cyborgs and always had access to the latest gadgets and toys. Amber, an absolute pioneer in computing, was everything I wanted to be: smart, awkwardly interesting and painfully in touch with all her feelings. Amber was also the owner of a set of Google Glass, the wearable technology that overlaid real-life data onto your field of vision.

In my estimation, that was exactly where I wanted to be. I didn't need a life with more apps to download, I needed a world with habits embedded in every nook and cranny of my life. Low screen to no screen was my goal.

Amber stumbled into the house, yodeling, "Helllllllooooo Chris!" I never failed to get excited to see her; she was a sister and a breath of fresh air all in one.

As usual, whenever she came packing technology, she was excited to show her new toy to me. I put the set on and was amazed. Here it was, September 2013, and I was walking around with a computer attached to my head, with a viewfinder laying information over everything I looked at. "Ok Glass," I said, and a menu dropped into my field of vision.

"Take a picture." Like magic, I could hear a camera click, and the image in front of my eyes was captured. "Ok Glass, what's the weather?" I could see the weather in front of me, both out the front window of our tiny home on Cherry Street and on top of the world around me through the clear lens of the Google Glass.

It dawned on me that if I could use Google Glass to constantly collect information on the world around me, then somehow send me urgent updates when I needed them, I could essentially unlock turn-by-turn directions, so to speak, for life's hard choices.

By the holidays in 2013, I had started using Google Glass to send me alerts when I hit a certain spending threshold while at a mall. It was just like my bar adventure, except this time I would create a rule that said if I spent more than $200 at the mall, I would receive an alert telling me to slow down. Like clockwork, as I strolled through Cherry Creek Mall, shopping for Christmas gifts with my newly minted exit cash from BMC, Google Glass sent me an alert: "Shop less!"

"Shop less." It was so simple. Again, location meets spending meets behavior. The remarkable thing about how we all manage our finances is that we so often miss a vital detail. How we spend our money shows us not only symbolically who we are, but also what we value.

WALGREENS WANTS YOUR PRESCRIPTIONS AND YOUR DATA

The proliferation of club cards, loyalty programs and frequent-shopper points all will show you the value of your behavior, finances and life, but in this case, this information is tied up behind the coupons you are offered. Trust me, the data in your loyalty cards is worth more than you will ever understand. It could even save your life. (No, I am not kidding.)

Not long ago, I stood onstage with the chief data scientist for Walgreens on a digital health panel. This gentleman strolled back and forth across the stage, telling a group of digital health experts how he had single-handedly created a Fitbit-like device that monitored Walgreens' balance rewards program members and helped them walk their way to a healthier life. How? By offering them discounts and special offers based on what Walgreens had learned about them.

My mouth was on the floor listening to this corporate puppet smugly detail how Walgreens owned all this consumer data and was supposedly making people better just by visiting "the corner of healthy and happy."

I was up next. "Let me get this straight. You monitor your customers' footsteps, prescriptions, all their purchases and then use this data to offer them discounts?" With a certain amount of glee in his eyes, the scientist nodded.

"I am not sure you should be that excited about turning people into walking coupons." The audience erupted in laughter. I went on to explain my concerns to the audience.

If Walgreens really cared about me, wouldn't it try to feed that information back to me, my health-care provider or even my family? Wouldn't it be more useful for me to understand my own health conditions and how my purchases could contribute to my well-being? Of course not, because that's not how corporations work. They live to make money off of our poor choices; making us healthier doesn't actually accrue to their bottom line.

What I am trying to say here is simple: where you spend your money is probably the single biggest factor in your emotional health. And we are letting corporations profit off of this knowledge, while we remain mostly ignorant of it.

In a cashless society, the quantified self belongs to banks, subscription services and loyalty programs, so until Elon Musk invents a bitcoin powered by sunlight here are three tips to help you and your family survive a post-cash society. Don't unplug.

MONEY TIPS

✦ **BEWARE OF STORED CREDIT CARDS:** The digital economy and its invisible appendages could be wrecking your financial life.

✦ **DIGITAL MASLOW:** Apply Maslow's hierarchy of needs to your digital finances and time to understand who you are and what you value.

✦ **PAYING WITH E-MOTIONS:** Split your payments between your wrist, bank and phone.

BEWARE OF STORED CREDIT CARDS

The digital economy and its invisible appendages could be wrecking your financial life.

As far as I can measure, your unseen optional spending— not on vital things like rent, utilities, food and so on—falls mainly into three areas: convenience spending, stored credit cards and subscriptions. Figuring out what's going on with the unseen money is the key to getting a handle on who and what you are online. While a majority of the sites that eat away at your time and attention are free, as in you're-the-product free, the sites, apps and services you buy that save your payment method, allow you to subscribe or don't require you to think before you purchase things are slowly draining your bank account dry.

You can feel it if you stand still for a moment and think about the ticktock of the Netflix account that you haven't been using since you finally polished off *Breaking Bad* two years ago. Or the annual subscription to Microsoft Office, dusty on the digital shelf of your laptop. That online HBO subscription that you forgot the password to after last season's *Game of Thrones* finale. The Amazon Kindle Unlimited subscription that you haven't used since you finished the last Harry Potter.

The first thing you need to do is measure your convenience spending each month. I need you to create a category or tag in your budget or accounting software for every dollar you spend that you can't *actually touch*, as well as any dollars you spend on things where you never see your cash or your credit card being used. Anything that can be considered what I call convenience spending, tag #invisible. Uber and Lyft rides: #invisible. Ordering food online and paying the extra delivery fee: #invisible. Take a few hours and review your spending for the last month. How much did you spend on things you can't physically show me right now? Big items like renting an apartment don't count; we are looking for uniquely digital connections.

Next up, stored credit cards. List all the services that have your credit card information saved: iTunes, Amazon, Google Checkout, PayPal, your browser itself, maybe your ex-spouse. Understanding where these cards are and how you access them is critical to understanding the invisible puppet lines to your financial life online. I bet a large percentage of that list is tied up in your invisible purchases. After all, Uber doesn't work until you enter your credit card information and save it on their server.

If you forced yourself to retype in your credit card number every time you wanted to buy something online, rather than saving it online or allowing your browser to do so, you would naturally, without even noticing it, start to spend less money online. Try to un-memorize your credit card number while you're at it. I've found that having to get up and go find my wallet when I'm slumped on the couch shopping online late at night is an excellent spending deterrent.

Finally, take a moment to research backward one year and find all your subscription services, such as apps that you pay for only once a year or digital services that have an annual billing cycle, and list them. These subscription-based apps are insidious, as you don't feel the monthly pain of them. Apple and Google allow you to see all your app-based subscriptions, but they don't make it easy to cancel or maintain this list.

Do you pay for Tinder Gold? Yeah, that's an invisible good. Do you pay for Amazon Prime shipping once a year? Doesn't everyone? How much of your yearly income is tied up in automatic subscriptions?

After an audit of the three digital arteries to your financial heart—convenience spending, stored credit cards and subscriptions—what do you think? Is it out of control? Can you see where convenience might be bankrupting your financial security? Good. Now do something about it.

DIGITAL MASLOW

Apply Maslow's hierarchy of needs to your digital finances and time to understand who you are and what you value.

The challenge with living in a digital world is applying real-world principles to the bits and bytes of life. Money doesn't buy happiness online any more than it ever did in real life. There must be a better way to understand all these invisible connections to your wallet.

Now that you have a comprehensive list of invisible transactions, stored payments and subscriptions, it's time to understand the digital identity you have built for yourself. Even if you don't do this exercise for your financial peace of mind, consider doing it for your mental health by examining the same things through the lens of time online. This exercise might just blow your mind.

If we go back to Abraham Maslow's hierarchy, start thinking about it in terms of your financial life. First level: physiological needs, things our bodies need to survive—food, clothing, shelter. Actually, these things are usually the easiest to define in a budget, so adding a category or a tag to these kinds of line items in your budget is pretty easy. How much money or time do you invest each month in items that are related to your physiological life? The old trope of spending no more than one-third of your salary on rent or housing lives on this level.

Next level: safety. Safety is defined as the things that help support our peace of mind. Financial safety is one category, and health and well-being are another. Health insurance is invisible and goes in here, but so does a subscription to Quicken, the popular online financial software. How much money or time do you spend a month focusing on safety items?

After safety, we get to the middle of the pyramid: social belonging. Social belonging refers to all the things related to relationships and intimacy. Time on Facebook, money spent on Tinder Pro. What about time spent texting?

The thing that blew me away the first time I applied Maslow's hierarchy of needs to my digital life was that a majority of my time was going to this level. (Interestingly, the majority of my *money*, though, was going to the top levels.) Think about it: How much money do you spend on your relationships? If the majority of your relationships are conducted mainly via Facebook, then you have a zero-dollar investment, but you probably have huge time costs.

Next up, we get to the really, really sticky level of esteem. I say this because the higher we transcend on Maslow's hierarchy, the stranger and more difficult seeing your digital doppelgänger can become. Esteem refers to the items in life we spend time or money on that support the story we tell about ourselves.

How in the world do you even wrap your head around that category? Well, for starters, time spent on social media consuming is different from time spent on social media creating. When we post to social media, we are creating an esteem budget. When we purchase a vacation, that probably belongs in the esteem bucket rather than the physiological needs bucket.

The dollars we spend on esteem services can be hard to track because our ego will fight the idea it's being fed. Our digital ego bleeds helplessly into the masses we connect to online. For me, I noticed that my esteem bucket was filled with items like my monthly website cost or my cell phone service from Verizon over the equally capable Sprint. Esteem budget items are items that support the story we tell ourselves about how important we are. As you evolve and become more intimate with who you are online and how digitally connected you are, you will find this category is a wild and woolly world of scary self-realizations.

The last stop on the original five layers of Maslow's hierarchy of needs is self-actualization. Self-actualization refers to becoming who you feel you are meant to be. (I have often thought that if my esteem category were truly in check, my self-actualization category would be the person I had already *become*.) I wasn't there yet, but for me, my goal was to become digitally well-rounded. A yearly subscription to Audible, the audiobook service, might be attributed here if you use that service to read widely and thoughtfully and better yourself. If your desire is to be the best partner or parent, then time focused on or money spent improving yourself in those categories would be applied to this bucket.

So how much money are *you* spending on each level? How much time do you spend each month in these areas? If your budget is out of whack and you need to save a few dollars, no problem. Start removing services and purchases from the top, self-actualization, down to the bottom, layer by layer. You'll find it is pretty easy to justify your spending at the bottom, but it gets harder and harder the higher up you go on your own personal hierarchy of needs.

Our digital lives are a series of connections that build a complex story, one that is algorithmically controlled by the service providers and time brokers in the world. Once you start to see all these connections, connections that are controlled by corporations not *you*, you might start to make different decisions.

PAYING WITH E-MOTIONS

Split your payments between your wrist, bank and phone.

For me, quantifying money was never enough. Understanding how I spent my money was always the key.

One of the craziest things I did during my financial hacking period was to ask the question, did the color of my credit cards change the way I spent money? Turns out, it did. Credit cards that were cheap looking, yellows and golds, I tended to use less than cards that were rich looking: blues, blacks, deep silvers. At one point, in order to spend less, I considered getting a credit card with a bad photo of myself on the front, just so I would be too ashamed to hand it to a cashier. (Oh, the power of self-censoring.)

Now that we are nearing the end of the glorious 2010s, most people have access not only to debit and credit cards but also an array of gift cards, loyalty payments and digital tools. Amazon lets us keep cash in their system, and both Apple and Google encourage us to upload our credit cards to their servers so that we can effortlessly pull out our phones to pay for anything, anytime. Their goal is, I suppose, to turn us all into financial cyborg Harry Potters, waving our device-laden wrists and hands at terminals all around the world.

Every day there seems to be another way to pay your friends back for that short-term loan, split the lunch bill or cover that sweatshirt we stole from them. We are at the point where it's easier to have our self-driving car take us to the nearest Walgreens and wave our Apple Watch through the air to pay for a bottle of SmartWater than it is to take enough steps to find a public water fountain in the mall. Like every other digital life hack I've shared, this one takes the challenge of extreme financial surveillance and connectedness and turns it into a golden opportunity for learning and exploration.

Consider that your financial outlays fall into three categories: old-fashioned credit cards, your phone and your wearable device (Fitbit, Apple Watch or Google Watch) that pays for items with a wave of the hand.

Make the decision to keep a credit card in your wallet, a

separate credit card stored in your phone and a third and different payment method on your wearable device, perhaps a debit card. With purpose and conviction, place your favorite payment card, the one you find easiest to use, perhaps because it earns airline miles toward your dream vacation, on your Apple Watch. Take your second favorite card and place that in your phone's payment system. Finally, carry your least favorite card around with you—maybe just your debit card. Now go live your life!

Here is what you will find. Because many find it humbling, or even embarrassing, to pay with your wrist, you might find you spend a lot less. For some reason, for most people, there is a natural tendency to not want to use technology to pay for something in front of other people, nervous perhaps that you're cashing a check that your technology can't honor. Next, because not everywhere allows you to use Apple or Google Pay, you'll probably put less on the card attached to your phone. Your last resort, using actual cash from the physical debit card in your pocket will be something you'll find yourself avoiding. I am willing to bet your spending patterns will change, perhaps even profoundly.

The newly revealed data of your digital life, a result of all your reporting, tied to your analysis of how you actually use money in terms of Maslow's hierarchy of needs, will be eye-opening. You will become a cyborg superstar when it comes to managing your own financial life. As large corporations devise better and sneakier ways to remove more cash from our pockets in the coming decades, you will be well-equipped not only to plan for retirement but maybe even to upload yourself to the cloud and know exactly how you're going to pay for it!

PART FOUR

KNOWLEDGE
(2012–2014)

Health and Environment

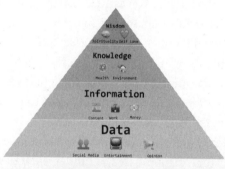

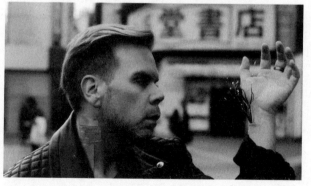

*Barbara Walters: "But what would you do if the
doctor gave you only six months to live?"*

Isaac Asimov: "Type faster."

What is knowledge? Is it something that comes from a textbook, a professor or a professional? Data lacks context; information needs some type of validation before it becomes knowledge. To understand how we travel from data to information and end up with knowledge, let's examine a GPS.

When you use a GPS, data is represented by the speed, direction and distance traveled. Those numbers don't factor into your starting point or your destination, they are just raw numbers. A map provides the platform to turn GPS sensor data into contextual information. You can see exactly where you are and all the data elements that are driving you.

If a GPS could understand historical trends and the future traffic of a highway, or if it could suggest when to leave so you have a more pleasurable time on the road, that would be more than information. Your GPS could be said to possess knowledge beyond the basic data that it is using.

This idea of mapping services being knowledgeable, rather than merely information-based, is fundamental to your understanding of the future of your connected life. All the large technology companies are creating mapping databases. Google and Apple don't care what you search for, they only care about where you are when you search and what they can offer to you at that time. Think of it as impulse buys at the grocery store, full time, everywhere. We are about to enter peak convenience when it comes to our consumer lives.

A map and a destination make the otherwise useless location sensors in your phone a knowledgeable system. Knowledge is the application of information systems over time to make their use more efficient for a certain goal. If your goal is to drive the fastest way on a route with no tolls or using back roads, the GPS becomes a knowledge appliance.

9

Health:
Don't Game or Shame Your Health

You Get Better by Taking Steps,
Not Counting Them

MEASURED TO DEATH

How many people do you know who have a Fitbit, Apple Watch or Samsung Gear on their arm? How many of your friends closely monitor their activity, sleep or food intake on their smartphone, or run with a heart-rate monitor strapped to their chest?

When someone is gravely ill in a hospital, no one questions the number of machines hooked up to them to check their respiration, heart rate or temperature. There's no shame in setting up an alert to go off when your heart decides it's time for an arrhythmia. Likewise, no one questions someone with diabetes who is obsessive about measuring their blood sugar levels. Instead, we think with relief, *Finally, it's about time.*

But today, people are slowly becoming immersed in systems that measure their entire biological life. How many babies are born into a life of full-time surveillance, with their parents constantly checking their breathing, movement, heart rate and sleep patterns online at all times of the day? I once counted 30 different digital solutions, from inception to age one, that a mom could put on, in or around her and her baby's body. We are birthing mini-cyborgs that are accustomed to constant health surveillance from the moment they start to breathe on their own.

If there is a cautionary tale in this book, it would come in the area of digital health, both what I learned about myself and, more urgently, what I learned by working in the industry of health insurance companies, physicians and wellness solutions. What I discovered about digital health and the upcoming monopoly on our wellness scares me deeply. We are living in a cult of wellness. The cult leaders are charlatans that believe if we give people enough incentives, they can will themselves to health.

The underlying argument at so many HR conferences these days is if we keep our employees healthy, they will be absent less and produce more. From insurance companies that give their members Fitbits and Apple Watches to large companies that have annual wellness days where people are measured, weighed and blood is taken, we live in a culture where if we can extract enough information, we think we can understand the risk pool.

It's hard not to feel like a piece of livestock when you look at our health-care system through this lens. This scares me because when you balance the current lack of affordable health care with the cult of measured wellness and apply a technical solution to it, you end up with a type of health-care Elysium.

Elysium, the 2013 sci-fi thriller starring Matt Damon, told the story of a world where the haves and the have-nots are not separated by wealth, power or privilege but instead by access to health care. For so many reasons, the cult of wellness and the absurdity of technological solutions to human problems seems like the perfect recipe for a thriller.

For a moment consider what life would be like if we applied the systems and methods I employed and the advice I have given to entire populations of people. Unfortunately, it looks hauntingly Orwellian—straight out of *1984*. So let us move cautiously as we lift our finger from the touchscreen and place the technology on or in our bodies full time.

AN APPLE A DAY SHOULD NOT NEED CHARGING

Since around 2012, your smartphone has been counting your steps even if you haven't been. In 2015, Apple decided that your health falls neatly into four buckets: nutrition, activity, sleep and mindfulness. It wasn't just Apple; Google has also been a pioneer in digital health with their Google Fit program. There is nothing new about digitizing your health—as far back as the late 1990s, Microsoft was creating a repository for your digital body called Health Vault.

Yet the evolution of the corporate battles over your health are darker and more twisted than a horror movie. Again, corporations are incentivized to keep people well, meaning tracked, measured, productive and at their desks. Each year since 2014, Apple's HealthKit has slowly introduced new health-care software platforms: CareKit and ResearchKit. I dare say that Face ID, the software that allows Apple to unlock your phone using facial-recognition techniques, will be used for mental health diagnoses at some point, if Facebook doesn't beat them to it.

What is digital health? We can trace its evolution back to 2007, when Gary Wolf and Kevin Kelly, a founding editor at *Wired* magazine, birthed a movement called "quantified self." This movement of IT geeks, academics and what can only be called the "worried well" took to their devices and technology to measure, understand and remedy their own health issues.

The idea of a quantified self is relativity simple: measure, understand and remedy your life using data. The items they focused on in those early meetings somewhere deep inside Silicon Valley were the strange places where behavior met technology.

Not sleeping enough? Create a spreadsheet for what time you go to bed and what time you rise. Now compare that data with the weather, and discover that humidity and air pressure are keeping you up at night!

Weight gain in the spring? No problem, track your food and travel schedule and find the hidden connections between increased carb and sugar intake during those conferences you attend every year in Vegas and those extra five pounds around your midsection.

These early digital life recipes gave way to the emergent biohacker movement sweeping the globe. Digital health, the quantified self, like much of this book, is about revealing the invisible world around you and possibly influencing your projected path.

Today, it seems like there is a Silicon Valley answer for everything. Need to quit smoking, drink more water, regulate your menstrual cycle, control your opioid abuse? Seriously, there's an app for that. At the root of all of these software solutions to our behavior lies the same foundation: surveillance, tracking and monitoring, along with a robust set of pattern-detection mechanisms.

There is an odd truism in our culture when it comes to our technologies and health that is impossible to miss once you're aware of it. We often treat our devices better than our physical bodies. Our phones are usually the latest version of whatever our favorite brand is, charged to a near-constant 100 percent, with up-to-date software patches, adorned in attractive or unbreakable protective cases and screen covers. They usually have some type of insurance coverage in case of damage, and we pay insidious, never-ending monthly fees to make sure all of their contents are backed up to the cloud daily, if not hourly.

Why do many of us protect the plastic, metal and glass hardware in our lives yet give so little money, attention or support to our own bodies—*our* hardware?

GAMING AND SHAMING THE SYSTEM

Understanding your behavior is key to making the changes that will start you on a journey of wellness and health, but because systems eventually change or are retired, you also need to understand your digital health future.

Yes, your Apple Watch and Fitbit can help get you up and moving, but most days, the last thing you want or need is another alarm vibrating on your wrist, letting you know another life system is on the cusp of failure, especially a system as important as your health.

Most people know instinctively that they haven't walked enough that day or slept well the previous night. We are also aware that our diet is likely a concoction of genetically modified, cancer-causing sugar and chemicals, designed to cheaply and easily get you through the rest of the day at work. No app or wearable can help you understand consequences better than the one you have between your ears, yet we are still slowly allowing ourselves to become dependent on nudges from technology.

I've met joggers who won't go for a run if their watch battery is dead. I've talked to swimmers that suffer massive regret if they don't measure their laps and dieters who walk away from their diet if they miss logging even one meal.

Our digital health lives are tied up in high-level game

theory. Game theory is a computational model used by designers to help us make decisions or "game" us into a choice. This massive cult of design is referred to by professionals in the technology space as "gamification." Fitbit badges and cheered-on weight-loss goals are good examples of gamifying our own battles with our health. Unfortunately, so much of our health care, when applied through the lens of gamification, feels a lot more like shame, or what I like to call "shamification."

Yes, it is motivational to see your weekly health statistics, but when they are also shown to everyone you work with, your family and your friends, you can feel ashamed rather than gamed. There are so many ways to help people get healthy with technology that would avoid this type of rampant society shaming, yet app designers and tech companies are lazy. They would rather have results that lead to increases in stock prices than actual happy customers.

Within a decade, *all* of our life's behavior will be backed up automatically by the devices that we wear on our bodies, keep in our homes, move us from place to place and monitor us at work. The three main health-care players globally in 2018—Apple Health, Google Fit and Samsung Health—will download sets of habits that connect to the mesh network of our existence and slowly condition us into new habits, giving us small nudges that change our behavior. We don't have app stores, we have habit stores; our homes are digital incubators, cybernetic Skinner boxes where we are slowly patched and upgraded.

Either way, your health in the future looks more like the IT department you live with today; the doctors and practitioners of the world of tomorrow look more like code jockeys than frumpy older men in white jackets with a stethoscope slung around their neck.

Let my story and tips be a guide and, at times, a cautionary tale to get yourself healthier, one download at a time.

VITALS 2008

When I turned 40 in October 2008, three different outpatient drug and alcohol rehab programs had "graduated" me. On weekends, while many people were surfing Facebook, you could find me trolling the internet's one-stop shop for hypochondriacs, WebMD. When not learning about what diseases I might have, I spent time in chat groups for people with diseases, on sites like Patients Like Me, figuring out what I would come down with next. Social networking for me was more about finding out possible ways to catch ailments than finding new ways to like Beyoncé.

My weight was close to 300 pounds, my BMI was nearly 40 and I was checking my blood sugar once a week. I took two different heart medicines for arrhythmia, plus blood pressure meds and thyroid meds. On any given day, I was drinking two to three 12-packs of Diet Coke, smoking two packs of Marlboro Light 100s and eating around 3,000 to 4,000 calories.

I had never tasted a salad. I had never put watermelon, oranges or grapes in my mouth. My optional vegetables at all meals for the first 40 years of life had been either corn or potatoes. I would order two large drinks at the fast food drive-through to, wink wink, hide the extra sandwiches as if I was ordering for two people. I wasn't imaginative in my eating— Chinese, Indian, Mexican meals never crossed my lips. My food list was limited to burgers, pizza or breaded chicken patties.

My personal relationships were horrible. Medicated for depression and anxiety, thousands of hours and dollars in therapy. I have to pause for a moment and ask, in the United States in 2008, was I symbolic of our world-class health-care system? Was this the best we could do?

After the two years I'd spent studying the digital connections of my social media, entertainment, opinion, work life and finances, it was time to take on the far larger threat to my well-being: my health.

How could my health and behavior data create a knowledge graph of supported beliefs so I could hack my sense of well-being? Was there something beyond calories? Was my eating influenced by where I ate, how much I spent, who was with me? I would soon find out, definitively: yes, yes and yes.

TIME TO CYBORG UP

I was collecting massive amounts of software-related data about my life and behavior. I had recently starting putting everything I ate into an online food diary called Lose It! My Fitbit was with me all the time, my phone was checking in and collecting more bits and pieces of information and it was all being diligently saved into my Google calendar in the background.

While no one in my life knew about my multiyear data project yet, I was about to double down by attending the 2012 Quantified Self Conference at Stanford University in Palo Alto. My multiple failed attempts to share my secret passion project with prominent people in the field of technology and science had been a flop. My results were real, the data was visible, yet my attempts to connect had fallen mostly on deaf ears. I was starting to feel like that aspiring singer who keeps getting turned away at the stage door while belting out a few bars to a star heading for their limo. If only my heroes could see what I had created, how it was changing me and what could be accomplished if we could harness the power of our phones for our health rather than ad sales.

For the Quantified Self Conference, I had written to the organizers and asked if I could present, but I had been denied. Instead I attended as a regular person. The weather on September 15, 2012, on the Stanford campus was brisk, and the sounds of students buzzing around the campus filled the air. The first session I attended was with the current king of biohacking, Dave Asprey, the self-proclaimed bulletproof executive—the guy who invented putting a stick of butter in your coffee. He was standing in the corner of a room with about 12 people, talking about how he was sending electrical currents through his head to hack his brain. From there I attended a few of the main sessions, where speakers stood onstage and gave their normal pitch: this is what I did, this is how I did it and this is what I learned—the three-legged stool of the quantified self.

In the expo hall, I picked up the first two wearables that would radically change my life. The first device was called a BodyMedia armband, just out from a new startup at the time, which unobtrusively collected galvanic skin response, motion and a host of other data points throughout my day and night. Several times a day, I would open the app on my phone, press a button on the armband and a small alert would sound as my behavior was uploaded to my phone. (I always felt like I was beaming up when I heard the sound, just like the rhythmic sounds of the 90s modem that connected me to CompuServe, AOL and Netscape.)

In the app, my behavior was highlighted brilliantly. Sleeping and moving were no longer just binary operations. There were dimensions to my data I had never seen before. I had sleep stages, I had activity levels—walking was not, in fact, the same as exerting myself. I started to understand what truly feeling rested meant by looking at the data behind the total hours of sleep.

The second piece of technology I purchased was a Zeo headband. Zeo was a wearable headband you used while you slept, like a Fitbit for your dreams. Where the BodyMedia did a great job of measuring my sleeping body, the Zeo would let me see my sleeping mind.

MASHING MOMENTS OF DATA INTO PHOTOS

I had turned into a simple data-collection machine, walking, sleeping, eating. One day while out walking, a track by Sade called "Pearls" came onto my Spotify, a torch song about relentless poverty in Africa. A quiet peace fell over me, as if I knew how to get ahold of my life and bad behavior. I stood in the morning cold for a moment, astonished at the profundity of how connected my life was, then started walking again. We all have these aha moments, the ones we don't race to Facebook to share. (Although I was going to.)

The music filled my ears over the quiet hush of my tree-lined neighborhood. As I looked out at the recently snow-covered roads of Park Hill in Denver, it dawned on me that I could make these changes whether I was tracking or not tracking. The difference was that I needed to believe that it was *me*, not the mounting piles of equipment making these changes.

With that, I snapped a photo of the moment and posted it to Instagram. But before I did so, I used two other apps to overlay information on my moment. First was the weather: feels like 31. Next was the location: Park Hill Library. Finally, the music: "Pearls," Sade. That photo, replete with all those pieces of information to quantify this ephemeral moment, made me proud. I posted it, with a Sutro filter from Instagram, to share this digital moment, feelings and all.

That photo still sits on my Instagram account, a reminder of not just a snowy neighborhood day but also the massive amounts of data influencing me—from my activity, to the weather, to the music filling my ears. That photo was the turning point in a process of moving beyond data to explore the wisdom behind moments of insight and clarity.

Long before Facebook allowed people to dislike or love posts, long before Snapchat would let us post the weather, the speed of our car or the place we were visiting on our posts, I was already mashing up data and life and sharing it on Instagram. What I learned about my life from these simple photos changed me.

For instance, a few weeks after my walk to Subway on that snowy April day, I took some screenshots of my meals at Subway. My heart was beating 77 beats per minute, my total walking time was 24 minutes, the sandwich had 9 grams of fat, Madonna was playing on my headphones, and the temperature inside the restaurant was 75 degrees. Once again, these data-filled snapshots started to reveal very clear patterns.

MONEY AND FOOD

In the beginning of 2012, I was far from the salad-eating, water-consuming Buddhist vegan I would evolve into by 2016. Back then, the idea of not eating at McDonald's every day was beyond anything I could cope with. So I made a simple deal with myself: If the meal was under $5, I had to walk to it. If the meal was under $8, I had to at least ride a bike. But if the meal was over $10 per serving, I was allowed to drive to it. Yes, $5 at McDonald's meant a 20-minute walk, an $8 meal at Subway meant a bike ride of about 30 minutes, and if I picked a restaurant like Chipotle, which was further away and ingredient-wise, a little healthier, I was allowed to get in my car. Some people sing for their supper; I had to sweat for my lunch.

After I purchased my first bike in May, I decided Chipotle would require a bike ride also. It was a 30-minute bike ride in both directions, and if I was about to consume 600 calories in tacos, this would be just the trick to move my health into high gear. I was thrilled. My categories—spending, activity levels, consumption, entertainment and media—were all starting to, essentially, talk to one another.

JAILBREAKING FOR DATA

What about social media? I was hopelessly addicted to Facebook and Twitter between 2012 and 2014. What if Facebook and Twitter could actually conspire to make me healthier? I loved Twitter; I loved the attention and feedback from Facebook; and binge-watching my friends' lives and stalking my coworkers was a favorite pastime. But I tended to participate in this guilty pleasure while sitting down—in fact, more often than not, I was actually lying down. What if my guilty-pleasure apps, like Facebook and Twitter, only worked while I was working out? Like the TV attached to a treadmill, could I find a way to only allow myself to use these services if I were moving?

In 2013, I found a very useful jailbreak for my iPhone. Jailbreaks are illegal changes to your mobile phone's operating system to give them functionality the manufacturer doesn't intend them to have. Now my phone's apps, such as Facebook, Instagram and Twitter, were unusable unless I was moving. (Today, Apple uses this type of technology in their phones—you can actually have your phone automatically text people when you're driving to alert them that you are busy so you don't get distracted.)

This changed my relationship to social media instantly and bound it forever to my activity levels for the day. The phone's GPS and accelerometer sensors locked my phone away unless I was out for a walk, ride or drive. Overnight all my social media use became exercise. (Often, I felt like a rat on a wheel, trying to get my fix, but in drastic times, you have to resort to drastic measures.) The hack didn't work very consistently or for very long, and having a jailbroken phone creates a host of other problems, but by simply modifying the phone's base behavior, I was forced into creating new habits. My social media was, for the first time in my life, helping me get healthier.

✦ ✦ ✦

All the data was coming together in a perfect storm; I was creating my own digital ankle bracelet. What about cigarettes? Could I finally figure out how to cut back on my smoking or quit entirely by using data? Marlboro Light 100s were my best friend, and there was no emotional problem that a new pack of cigarettes didn't solve for me.

I loved to smoke so much that I would actually make myself sick by late afternoon each day. Most days, around 2 p.m., as I was consuming somewhere between my fifteenth and twenty-fifth can of Diet Coke, I would light up my thirtieth cigarette of the day. I knew intellectually that there was no way I could lose all the weight I needed to unless I cut back on smoking, so I had to figure out what triggered me.

As usual, I turned to my data. Hmm. This was a problem. Getting into the car was a trigger. Eating was a trigger. Friends who smoked were triggers. Beer was a huge trigger. Were there any behaviors that made me not want to smoke or at least smoke less?

Then I found it. For some reason, if I drank a lot of water, I smoked less. I looked deeper. It also seemed that the more I ate, the more I smoked. What if the meal was just an excuse to get to the cigarette? Was I eating more than I needed to simply to provide an excuse to smoke afterward? As it turned out, that was exactly what I was doing.

I also found that if there was a Diet Coke in one hand,

there tended to be a cigarette in the other. But if I wasn't drinking Diet Coke, I barely lit up.

Armed with this new information, I started binge-smoking, then drinking massive amounts of water. The idea was to try to link that feeling of a tight chest and sore lungs to liquid overconsumption. I wanted to create a connection between two seemingly separate activities, to train my brain to hesitate before lighting up. Indeed, the two became so inseparable that I naturally started slowing down the cigarettes when I drank tons of water, which in turn led to me actually eating less. I'm probably one of the few people I know who actually lost weight when they smoked less and then finally quit altogether.

We are so often told things about our bodies and our health, but we are rarely given the tools to create the kinds of connections that facilitate true understanding of ourselves. To this day, when I meet smokers, I tell them to drink more water, and to smoke before they eat instead of after, assuring them that this tactic will get them to lose weight as well as eventually quit smoking. As it turns out, the connections between the data are far more important than the data itself.

PEEING IN THE MIDDLE OF THE NIGHT

With this much water consumption, I, no surprise, had to pee all the time. This led me to some fresh insights into sleep.

If there was one thing I didn't need data to understand, it was that changes in my sleep schedule affected everything from my mood to my ability to exercise. I just needed to figure out how to fix it.

I started posting my sleep stats to Facebook to begin to mine my own data. Slowly, my sleep stats started filling up my timeline: 8 hours sleep, 9 hours sleep, 12 hours sleep, 3 hours REM sleep, 2 hours deep sleep.

Once I looked at the mountains of correlated data, I could see what was working and what wasn't. There was one glaring thing that was keeping me up in the middle of the night, and it was something we all face from time to time: having to pee.

I knew it would be simple enough to sort out a solution, but first I needed to figure out what drove the behavior. Of course, I could cut back on drinks before bed, but that seemed both unlikely and not focused enough for me.

I wanted to be precise—I'd rather know exactly what to cut back on and at what time. So I put Wemo sensors near my fridge in the kitchen. The Wemo sensor is a simple motion sensor that logs an incident every time it senses someone's movement. If I only got drinks from the fridge, then I could have a good idea of the window of time in which I consumed fluid. The next sensor I needed was to monitor the exit of said fluid. Yup, I needed to record when I peed, so I mounted a second Wemo sensor by my bathroom toilet. I had created a simple feedback loop to help me capture things going in and coming out of my body. Also, I wanted to find out if there was a difference in how I spent that time or what exactly I drank.

For weeks I changed my consumption patterns: more in the morning, less at night, more in the afternoon, nothing after midnight, nothing after 9 p.m., water, Diet Coke, beer. I logged what I consumed and when it came out. My goal was to sleep through the night for eight straight hours without having to pee. And after a few weeks, I managed it.

The secret formula wasn't complicated at all: no caffeine after 3 p.m., no water after 7 p.m. Water went through me fastest, and I never eat and drink water at the same time. I could have as much of anything else I wanted the rest of the day, even a caffeine-free Diet Coke before bed, but if I stuck to this method, I would sleep a full eight hours without having to pee.

HACKING SLEEP

Next I wanted to improve the quality of my sleep. I started experimenting with sound and sleep to figure out how to put myself in a deeper sleep so I could wake up more rested. Just like some people are side sleepers while others are back sleepers, some people prefer silence as they fall asleep, as opposed to a musical dream track. For the most part, I had never slept in a quiet room. If I wasn't listening to music, I needed white noise, preferably a fan, but what I didn't understand until I started logging was what the fan noise really was. Fan noise has a decibel level of 67 to 71, with a beats per minute of close to 50.

For me, sleep, that elusive demon, was critically important, and getting my mind ready for bed was a full-time job. To combat my racing mind, I started consuming audiobooks. Falling asleep is pretty difficult when you have 800 milligrams of caffeine from 20 cans of Diet Coke in you. But what's better than a boring book to put you to sleep? Putting audiobooks on a one-hour timer usually did the trick. For me, the voice had to be male, preferably British. (Listening to Winston Churchill's *A History of the English-Speaking Peoples* cured a lot of insomnia.)

And what about music? Could I create a playlist to make me sleepy? Could I condition myself, like Pavlov's dogs, to go to sleep?

While there was a bit of Jedi mind trickery involved, I found out that yes, it certainly was possible. I started with a baseline assumption: if I could learn to sleep to certain music, by extension, certain music could probably lull me into being sleepy. To do this, I needed to train my mind with music, but up until this point, listening to music, unlike books, tended to keep me awake.

I decided the best plan would be to schedule specific music

to play in the middle of the night. It wasn't easy at first to figure out the decibel level. How loud was too loud, which would
serve only to wake me up? How soft was too soft, so that my
body wouldn't be able to sense the beat? I knew that there was
something pretty odd about telling your Sonos to start playing
music at 4 a.m., but I really believed that this hack might improve my sleep. I wanted to have music start and stop while I
was sleeping in order to teach my mind what it was like to be
in a dream state.

It took weeks of conditioning, but scheduling a very precise
Enya playlist or gentle piano music to come on in the middle
of the night, approximately three hours after I fell asleep, allowed me to stay asleep and improve the quality of that sleep.
To this day, upon hearing the first few notes of "Boadicea" by
Enya, I feel like I've just had a Klonopin with a rum-and-Coke
chaser.

Once I had figured out what music helped me sleep better,
the next trick was to have my sleep playlist start playing hours
before my bedtime at a very low level, in order to start to slow
me down. While all this might seem like a bit much, if you've
ever had even garden-variety insomnia, you know that you'd
bite off your arm and write a book on the wall with your bloody
stump to get some sleep.

I didn't just use sound to help my body prepare for sleep;
I also focused on how lighting could help or hinder my healthy
sleep patterns. Using a series of Hue smart lights, I created a
slow, cascading mood shift in my basement warren. It started
at sundown and gradually dimmed over the course of the evening, changing the tone of the lights from amber to deep purple.

In the morning when it was time to get up, my lights would
slowly start turning on, shifting from complete darkness to a
pale pink color. Enya would also start playing slowly; the same

artist who had peacefully sent me into slumber also brought me into the world each day.

My sleep soon became deeper, more restful, more restorative. Nine-hour nights of sleep with at least 50 percent of that time spent in deep or REM sleep became common. Sleeping more and better changed how I lived my waking hours profoundly. As I shared all my sleep hacking insights online, my friends actually became much more interested in my life. They didn't care about my attempts to become more active, but I had a hunch that being a world-class sleeper might impress them. And I was right. Everyone cares about sleep.

While a lot of people post their runs and workouts to social media nowadays, for me, switching to just posting good nights of sleep was enough to create the sort of feedback loop that would set me up for a better day. I knew my friends would like me if I was getting more sleep, so I changed my patterns and habits in order to do so—positive reinforcement helped cement new patterns.

Just 20 minutes more of REM or deep sleep and I could increase my activity from walking one hour to jogging for 30 minutes. Going to bed earlier and faster meant I spent less time watching TV and playing around on the web. When I didn't participate in those types of evening activities, which I had already seen tended to lead to unhealthy behavior for me, it allowed me to focus more on my health the next day.

If you are having problems today, I can almost guarantee you that the problems actually started last night while you were (or weren't) asleep. The challenge with sleep today is that we tend to get so little, we often wake up already dreading how we will feel that day. The dread continues throughout the day, and by the time we get into bed, it's too late. We have set ourselves up for another night full of tossing and turning.

Challenging as it may be, what we need to do is capture

what good sleep looks like—environment, temperature, light, scents, sound and so on—and then recreate it as often as possible. Does this fix insomnia outright? Some sleep scientists would say no, but I can promise you that it helps move you forward. All you need is a few good nights of sleep to see the light at the end of the tunnel.

As I became more and more maniacal about my sleep and exercise patterns, I discovered another dark side to data-logging. If you miss data, it's almost as if the sleep or exercise didn't count. I remember one day I headed out with my latest Fitbit on my wrist to take a walk. After several minutes of walking, I realized that my Fitbit was dead. I was furious, realizing that all the steps I was taking weren't going to "count."

BEYOND SLEEP DATA, ARE YOU A WEREWOLF?

Then Sleep Cycle showed up on the market. Unlike other sleep-logging apps of its day, it was deceptively simple. Created by a Swedish man who traveled a lot and wanted a better way to log his sleep and wake up in the morning, the app utilizes the accelerometer, gyroscope and GPS on your phone. When you placed it next to you on your bed, it tracks your movements throughout the night.

What I loved about this app was the graphic component. Seeing my movements at night helped me understand so much more about my sleep. Sometimes I would go out like a light, as my mother used to say, and for the first time, I could actually see it represented beautifully, right there on my phone. The graph would have a nice high awake level, then boom, within moments that line would swoosh to the bottom of the graph and just mildly undulate for the next seven to eight hours. It was oddly satisfying to wake up feeling well rested and be able to corroborate that feeling by seeing my stillness in bed on the app.

Sleep Cycle also logged all sorts of other environmental factors, such as location, weather, even moon cycles. Who knew, but it turned out that full moons wreak havoc on my sleep. According to an employee of Sleep Cycle I met years later, this is actually a large factor for many women, but only a small percent of men are affected. Why don't most sleep apps tell us about the moon cycle, weather or environmental factors? It would be helpful to give us something to blame other than ourselves for our poor nights of sleep. Using the app, I started planning my sleep around the full moon. I also learned that I slept like a bear during good weather, but on rainy days, I might be sleepy, but I wasn't getting good sleep. More and more, I was starting to see the abundant connections not only between my data and my behavior, but also the connections with the world around me.

EXERCISE AND SLEEP

Another feature that taught me a lot about how I spent my days and how it affected my nights was a simple quiz that I created in Sleep Cycle. Each night, when I set my alarm, I'd answer a few questions, such as what type of workout I had done that day, whether I was going to sleep listening to music or not, whether I was traveling, had meditated and so on.

You don't need Dr. Oz to tell you that a bit of movement during the day will help you get a better night's sleep, but it's not that simple. For me, at the beginning of my health kick in 2012, movement, which took the form of walking, was hard. I would come home after only 20 minutes, legs sore, mind confused, out of breath and worried I would never get better. But by 2014 I was sleeping better. I had gone from hardly walking to hitting the gym a few days a week and even going for a run occasionally. Yet, some days, when I thought I'd done everything right, my sleep was terrible. How could this be?

As it turned out, overdoing it was my problem, at least some of the time. It's counterintuitive to lay off a good thing though, so I wanted to take a closer look. For me, whenever I hit 20,000 steps, my sleep would be 30 percent less efficient (as measured by movement while I'm in dreamland).

This was staggering to see, and it created its own set of challenges. For example, if I was out of town or in a foreign country on vacation, I couldn't just stop walking midway through the day. Worse yet, on travel days, airports can really boost your step count. So I initiated plans on travel days and even walking days to actually skip the steps using escalators and elevators in order to save myself from going over that critical 20,000-step mark.

Now let's be honest, many of us will never make the bullshit necessary 10,000-steps-a-day metric that is sold to us by the big-data pushers of the digital health world. I did a lot of research into sleep and talked to various sleep scientists to prove this to myself, but it makes sense to experiment with your own window of possibility, to find out whether a limit of 4,000 or 14,000 steps might help you increase your sleep quality.

Another thing to watch for with sleep is the type of training you're doing. At the gym, trainers encourage you to mix it up, which usually means alternating cardio and strength training. Something they don't tell you is how the different types of training affect your sleep.

We all have read that just 30 minutes of exercise a day can have a profound effect on our mood, but is it that simple? Is there more to learn? Does it need to be a certain type of activity? Are walking, lifting weights or even short sprints all created equal?

By logging the types of activity I did during the day, I was able to see when and how it had an impact not just on my day, but also my nights. Net fitness trackers tell you to get 30 minutes of exercise. Some people just make that cumulative. What I found was that you needed 30 minutes of continuous movement to make a change. If you want your 10,000 steps to make a difference, you'll do 30 percent of them at once—in other words, take a walk of 20 minutes or more. But try to avoid a long walk after dinner or before bed. Activity is required for an excellent night of rest, but too much activity near bedtime will disturb your rest—as will engaging in certain types of activity. For instance, if I was at the gym doing normal strength training, meaning working with resistance and weights, I would sleep significantly deeper and better than if I had spent that time on a treadmill doing cardio training.

The solution was simple: On days where there were other sleep stressors—stress, anger, caffeine, weather conditions, deadlines—I would make sure to do strength training at the gym. Days where everything else was good in my sleep world, I'd allow some cardio.

Perhaps if our gym life was more adaptive to our actual life, maybe we wouldn't hate the gym so much.

MEDITATION AND SLEEP

If you meditate, you will not sleep as well. This is the exact opposite of the promise of meditation. In my experience, meditation always dropped my sleep efficiency. I've speculated that this is happening because meditation does two things to us. First, it increases awareness of our thoughts. Think about that: What is the difference between early stage insomnia and meditation? After 11 p.m., failing to control a busy mind, well, that's what we call insomnia. If we try doing it at 6 a.m. or during an after-work yoga practice, we call it meditation.

There are different forms of mediation, and not all meditations are created equal. If you wish to sleep better, gratitude

practice or loving kindness is key. As you become more profi-
cient at meditation, you might see a decrease in insomnia
symptoms, but that brings us to the second feature of meditation: abandonment of attachment. That's a fancy way of saying
you've learned how not to worry, and let me tell you, meditation is the fastest way to this state.

The problem is, you learn that not sleeping is ok and part
of life, so guess what? You might sleep less. If someone had told
me at the beginning of my journey that meditation and exercise
would make sleeping *more* difficult, I would have laughed, as
that goes against all the wellness indoctrination in our current
society. More on meditation later, but suffice it to say, your sleep
is affected by almost every choice you make during the day.

As of right now, the little town of Kapa'a in Kauai was
where I got the best sleep of my digital life, followed closely by
Venice, Italy, and Frillesås, Sweden. If I wanted to sleep poorly,
I could go and hang out in Kyoto, Japan; Montreal, Canada; or
Helsinki, Finland, though to be fair, being in Kyoto was like
meditating full time. (Rather than being good for sleep, it was
pretty much an awakening of epic proportions.)

Sometimes there is nothing wrong with you, it's the world
that has an issue. You either need to learn to live with it or wait
it out. As for me, I'm a bit more cautious now with my sleep
and with all the data that goes along with it—it is helpful to
know a lot, but data, information and knowledge can't solve all
my problems. Like all of us, I still struggle from time to time
with my sleep, and all the advice and blame in the world doesn't
make it better. Sometimes you just need to be ok with imper-
fection.

At some point in the future you will be asked to measure
some aspect of your health. More than likely you will use your
phone to do so.

There are three simple rules to consider when looking at

your digital health. First, active, rested, calm or nourished—pick one. Second, don't get hurt by the numbers. And lastly, don't allow yourself to be reminded into bad habits.

Before someone else unplugs you, don't unplug yourself.

HEALTH TIPS

✦ **LIVE IN ONE CATEGORY AT A TIME:** Learning to manage your health in one of four areas (nutrition, activity, sleep and mindfulness) will let you focus on getting healthier.

✦ **YOUR HEALTH IS NOT A NUMBER:** Be careful when evaluating your health. Your habits are more than numbers to be hacked.

✦ **AUTOMATION IS ONE-SIDED:** Take reminders from health apps with a grain of salt and create dedicated spaces for them.

LIVE IN ONE CATEGORY AT A TIME

Learning to manage your health in one of four areas (nutrition, activity, sleep and mindfulness) will let you focus on getting healthier.

According to the scientists, designers and technologists at 1 Infinite Loop, Cupertino, CA 95014, better known as Apple, Inc., your health fits neatly into four areas. Log in to any smartphone app store and you will find your health divided into nutrition, activity, sleep and mindfulness. It's not a bad starting place if you would like to better understand how you're living your life.

Our phones are constantly collecting information about our lives, regardless of our privacy preferences, so understanding how digital health on your phone works can be key to understanding yourself.

No matter how I looked at the data, starting in one of these four quadrants kept leading to the others. Can't sleep? Perhaps you took too many steps today. Overeating during the holidays? Increasing your activity will curb the unwanted winter bulge.

Start small and only in one area. Don't try to tackle meditation, walking, eating better and going to bed early in one fell swoop. Yes, I know our devices make managing our health seem as easy as shopping, but it's not. Our bodies are elaborately complicated systems with dependencies you don't learn about until you uncover them.

For me, activity was a good place to start back in 2010. Just focusing on moving was enough in the beginning. Don't bother trying to eat perfectly if you have never eaten healthily in your life. Just focus on adding a little more action to your day. This doesn't even have to be walking—just standing counts as movement to our devices.

If activity really isn't your thing, then taking a look at nutrition might be easier. Start with logging your food. There are hundreds of apps that allow you to do everything from scanning barcodes to downloading meal plans. Software makers promise big data and artificial intelligence to design diets that will melt the pounds away, but I can promise you if you just skip French fries for a few weeks, you'll glory in some amount of success.

Maybe you live in a cold climate or don't have access to a lot of healthy options because of travel or budget? Then start with sleep. From my decade of logging thousands of behaviors and habits, there is no single more potent solution to health ills than a good night of sleep. Need to lose a bit of weight? Lose the jogging shoes and abandon your quest to eliminate energy drinks. Instead buy a good pillow and a quiet fan for your room. Seriously, an extra 30 minutes of sleep each night will melt away five pounds in less than 60 days.

One of the challenges with sleep, though, is the obscene amount of advice there is about how to get, keep and create quality slumber hours. Most sleep apps won't help you sleep better, but they can coach you into better environmental and behavior conditions to create the atmosphere for good sleep. The other more serious problem with sleep and digital health is the sheer ease with which we can pathologize our numbers. When you start measuring your sleep, it becomes far too easy to let seeing a five-hour night of sleep in your sleep app define everything you do from 9 a.m. to 7 p.m. that day. (More about judgment later.)

Finally, now that you have considered activity, nutrition and sleep, it's time to mention no one's favorite word, mindfulness. In a culture that places an inordinate amount of value on the importance of staying busy, encouraging someone to develop or explore a mindfulness practice doesn't seem like sound advice. There is an entire chapter dedicated to my spiritual pursuits later in this journey, but for now, let's keep it simple.

You don't need a meditation app to meditate. If you clean your house, drive a long distance to work or frequent extended meetings, you are probably meditating at that point. Meditation is merely the act of paying attention nonjudgmentally, moment to moment, to your thoughts. Sitting on a cushion and focusing on your breath is just a trick to get you to notice that your mind doesn't stop. It's only then that gurus tell you that the goal is not to stop your mind but to become ok with its ridiculous levels of activity as a calm observer.

No matter where you start with for your digital health, it's important to remember that these four areas—activity, nutrition, sleep and mindfulness—all work independently of each other. If you don't feel like running or meditating, hit the salad bar and climb into bed early.

Your phone is a gateway to a world of distraction or awareness. Start by looking at your relationship with your health as
a series of applications and decisions. Life doesn't need a resolution, it needs a good data plan.

YOUR HEALTH IS NOT A NUMBER

Be careful when evaluating your health. Your habits are more than
numbers to be hacked.

Our computers, phones and technology are often lumped under
the jumbled banner of digital. "Digital" actually just means
that something runs on 1s and 0s. Something is on or it's off.
In spirituality, there's a name for this: duality. If you ever wonder about the polarization in the world as we race into the
2020s, look no further than the fact that everyone you meet
is living in a system of yes or no. Computers don't have the
option to say maybe. "Fifty shades of gray" lives only in the
physical world.

For many people, learning to live by a number can be a real
lifesaver.

But life isn't digital, life is quantum—the step beyond digital where all possibilities happen at once. It's incredibly difficult to stick to a diet when you live with a family, step-counting
can feel like being bullied when you're visiting your aging parents, and sleep monitoring will ruin your mood for entire days
once you become too aware.

The challenge comes from our ability to define the par-
ameters in which we want to live: 10,000 steps, 8 hours of
sleep, 1,500 calories and 30 minutes of meditation, which butts
up against the real-world necessities of answering email and
not missing soccer practice.

My advice is simple: Don't look at numbers through the
lens of today, and never, ever look at your health data through
the lens of right now. Instead, use your digital health apps to

look at your life through the lens of at least a week. I prefer a month, but a week will work. Seeing trends over large periods of time will help you accomplish them.

The challenges of digital health and data can make you feel like a complete loser. If you're having problems sleeping, do not, I repeat, do not track sleep. And if you must track sleep, don't look at the number when you wake up!

Next, don't friend or connect to others on digital health apps until you are ready to feel compared, judged and shamed. Many health-care plans, employers and major technology companies proclaim the benefits of gamifying your health. Studies show you get great results when you are compared to your peers. Yet, this biological version of Facebook will leave you hating your friends, family and yourself. Do not friend anyone on a health social network when you are not feeling good about yourself.

Finally, before you blame yourself for your lapses and your perceived imperfections, look around. You will see in the next chapter that your environment plays a huge role in your health, and unless you measure both, you'll spend a lot of time blaming yourself.

AUTOMATION IS ONE-SIDED

Take reminders from health apps with a grain of salt and create dedicated spaces for them.

There is no shortage of people in the world reminding you to be healthier. We all know that fitness guru, always at the gym, encouraging us to take a walk or eat a salad or offering us the latest article on why we need to learn to meditate. Unfortunately, this also spills over to our devices. Ask anyone with a Fitbit or Apple Watch what it's like to have your arm vibrating, telling you to stand up, take a walk, go to sleep. Our cybergenetic

overlords bark orders at us and we respond like tethered pup-
pets on 4G strings.

The notifications you configure on your phone can be a
health program killer unless you are ready to have a terminator
overload. If you struggle with the concept of machines telling
you to get off your butt—and let's be honest, you should—then
you have some work to do before you start your digital health
journey. Consider turning off all alerts, popups, sounds and
app badges in your health apps in the beginning. They can feel
overwhelming, and they don't understand a lot of our lives.
The last thing you need in the middle of a dark theater is your
device telling you to get up and take a walk. Why do our cars
drive themselves, but our phones can't seem to fathom that getting the last 1,500 steps in probably isn't great life advice at 75
miles per hour at 11:47 p.m. at night?

Instead, most phones have an area where you can see a list
of missed alarms and alerts. On Google phones, you pull down
from the top; on Apple, the "today" screen is a swipe right.
Make this or any other dedicated place on your device the only
area where you get alerts about health, and consider removing
all other alerts from these areas. (It can feel horrible to see an
encouragement to get more sleep tonight right above three
phone calls from your boss at 8 p.m. checking on a work deadline.)

Finally, one of the often-neglected truths of digital health
is the complete and honestly shameful ignorance of the differences between sexes—our devices don't consider meno-
pause, pregnancy or ovulation when making suggestions to
us. Technology also doesn't take into consideration that you
are recently out of surgery or that you're suffering from a bout
of depression. Strangely enough, our technology is aware of all
of these circumstances—programmers just don't account for

them when programming decisions. But you have more control than you think over turning your phone into a kind and encouraging personal trainer instead of a malevolent health dictator.

10

Environment: Smart Homes Don't Care About You

All Bad Habits Come from Convenience

The way you interact with the world will change profoundly in the coming decades. As much as smartphones have changed our lives already, the Internet of Things (IOT) will disrupt things even more. IOT is loosely defined as anything without a screen that is attached to the internet, otherwise known as *smart*: smart homes, smart devices, smart buildings.

Social media and mobile phones have forever altered your attention; connected systems fundamentally changed your work life. In this same profound way, IOT will deeply influence your health. The challenges of IOT are ripe with FUD (fear, uncertainty and doubt), and pundits won't hesitate to scare you about privacy invasions, hacking or identity theft. And while I agree there are issues we need to worry about, as our refrigerators get sensors that scream at us to throw out the chicken, I believe that IOT will be invaluable in helping us focus on factors that influence our mood, health and life.

IOT exists all around us. For the most part, there's no screen to look at. So it's important to think about *why* we want to network everything in our homes, cars and workplaces. Does everything you buy need a connection to the internet?

IOT devices fall into two distinct categories: convenience devices that make life easier, and informant devices that speak to other devices.

Convenience devices, like smart speakers—Amazon's Alexa, Apple's HomePod, Sonos speakers and Google Home—make life easier. These voice assistant AIs, or artificial intelligences, listen for us, then send our requests off to the internet. Within seconds, answers are sent back to us. These assistants can do small tasks for us or even automate some tasks. Turn on the lights, order pizza, set a timer, play a song. Our phones do all these things too, but our phones require us to unlock our screens, download apps, pay attention to them and remember specific commands; they don't integrate into the air around us like IOT devices do.

The informants are devices that passively collect information in the background to tell us or other devices what's going on. For example, a mattress that collects your heart rate and respiration while you sleep, or the sensor that records the temperature, humidity and noise in your bedroom or the new refrigerator that keeps track of your foods' expiration dates.

Thousands of these types of devices are being created each day, and no matter how many new items we embed the internet inside of, the reality is that we are simply making it easier for machines to collect information about us.

Why is this concerning? As our lives become increasingly connected at work and at home, our decisions will be outsourced to our devices. In other words, our decisions will be taken away from us.

NO SCREEN, NO CHOICE

When you ask your smart speaker to read a book, you need to have a book on your smart speaker's servers, one that you likely have purchased from their parent corporation. That is to say, you better own this book, the one you're listening to right now, on whichever device you're connecting with. Amazon's Alexa doesn't care that you have books purchased from Apple, and Apple doesn't care that you pay for Spotify. If it's not making more money for their own corporation, the bottom line is that they won't help you. Because the ugly reality is that these devices' main goal isn't to make your life easier; it's to force you to live entirely within their own corporate ecosystem.

This is urgently important for people to understand. The roots of the digital arms race can be traced back to the mid-1990s when the Department of Justice took Microsoft to court because Bill Gates and his team wanted to integrate an internet browser into their desktop operating system. It seems silly. What difference does it make to have Internet Explorer's little blue "E" on every desktop, really? Who cares? But, in fact, it is of massive importance. Just as emails were filling our lives, the browser that opened when you clicked a link in them was about to be forced to Internet Explorer rather than the king at the time, Netscape.

Stop for a moment and think about the defaults in your life. By 2005, anyone over the age of 15 had been confronted with the question, "Do you wish to make XXXX your default browser?" Very few people think about how this setting has moved way beyond your internet browser.

By 2010, many people had been asked to pick a default mail app on their phone. Many of us will have multiple apps on our phones for email, one for personal and another for work. Most people have an overly scheduled life and need to pick a default calendar application.

Now our life is chock-full of defaults, and the impact of these seemingly casual decisions is something that keeps me up at night. Take a moment to think about something as simple as your default map applications. Maybe you like Apple Maps; perhaps you prefer Google's. But let's say you have a Tesla. Now you can't use either map because Elon Musk doesn't like those maps. (By the way, this is true.)

Just as Google defined the virtual world, big tech companies know that your applications give the physical world context. So if an ice-cream shop, dry cleaner or chain store isn't listed on the map of your default map applications, it doesn't exist.

In the next five years, many of you will start interacting with technology using your voice. Your defaults will be chosen for you by your habits. Your ability to navigate the world and understand your choices will be defined by the tech companies you use. More urgently, your access to services, people and tools will be defined by the relationships those tech companies have with other tech companies.

What are the default applications and hardware you've selected or purchased that are already dictating your life? Have you already locked yourself into something that you can't get out of? I fear we are headed toward a population of people lost in the real world because of decisions they've made in the virtual world.

Today, most people pay for content like Netflix, a music service, possibly a book service, and they use map apps, calendar apps, reminder apps and note apps. They have cooking apps, apps for counting steps, apps for banking and so on. If you ask an AI assistant to create a reminder, read a book or direct you to your mother-in-law's house, you better hope that reminder app works with your phone, car, home and laptop, that your book is on whichever service the AI runs, that your map program works in your car.

LET'S BE HONEST, YOUR HOME IS JUST AN EXPENSIVE IPHONE CASE

The promise of IOT for convenience is dangerous. You are ceding control to the ultimate boss in the data-plundering game of your life, and the devices that inform other parts of your life are getting swiftly locked down in a battle between what is essentially a small handful of massive corporations.

Your health, home and car are all about to be uploaded to the cloud. Don't believe me—try to buy a Fitbit and use it with an Apple iPhone. Very soon, your phone will know everything about where you are and how quickly you're getting there. Ask Google to tell your Tesla where to go. Have Alexa play a YouTube video for you. You can't! Your wishes are not their command. These companies don't have agreements with each other. The lines are drawn, your life is about to be a battleground, and in case you haven't noticed, you're paying $9.99 a month to 15 different providers to listen to the new Britney track at home, in the car and at the gym.

In the future, we will buy homes and cars based on the operating systems they run. Moving to a new house or city will be just like upgrading your phone—you'll take along your preferences and your data. The rest will be handled by the new house or car and their operating system.

As I started to measure the world around me and create routines to slowly chip away at my longest-running bad behaviors, it became obvious that the future of technology is in health and home. But until then, let's look at the world you might be missing right in front of you. Hey Siri, Ok Google,

Alexa, Cortana, read the next chapter to me and put on some Beck at 50 percent volume.

✦ ✦ ✦

The more I tracked, the more I realized all the things I *wasn't* tracking. I wanted to measure environmental factors at home, which I could control to a certain extent, and factors out in the world, which I couldn't.

Photos that were captured in my Google calendar were now augmented with the temperature, humidity, rainfall, air quality, sunrise, sunset, ambient noise levels, brightness and LUX levels. Suddenly, a whole unseen world around me was opening up. Rainy days and Mondays now made a lot more sense.

Do you remember the Carpenters? Or can you jump onto Spotify and stream some for me? Yeah, Karen Carpenter, who famously bemoaned rainy days and Mondays and their effect on our moods. Is there data to actually back that up? Much to my surprise, pop clichés and old wives' tales are spot-on more often than you'd think.

LISTENING TO MY BIG MAC

My desire to eat poorly didn't start or stop with exercise. To this day, even as the healthiest me I've ever been, I still dream of taking a dip in the chocolate river that runs through Willy Wonka's factory. To find a balance between my intake and my waistline, many more things had to evolve. I had already decided that eating at McDonald's was a necessity. If it took walking there, so be it. If I had to buy a bike to permit myself to eat a burrito at Chipotle, that's what I did.

But as I fell deeper and deeper into my data hole and carefully studied the places I ate, my understanding of fast food was evolving too. Let's start with some basics. Fast food is fast.

It is made quickly, it is served quickly and it is consumed quickly. One day, while eating my Filet-O-Fish—all 390 calories of it, made up of 40 percent carbs, 44 percent fat and 15 grams of protein—I happened to notice the speed with which I was devouring this sandwich, along with the small fries I had bought to keep me from going off the deep end and ordering a burger too.

So I put my headphones on and started listening to some music. Deep forest and the ambient jungle sounds of 90s trance music transported me. Suddenly I was chewing more slowly and enjoying my food more. What was going on?

Although I conducted several experiments with food and music, I couldn't figure out exactly why I was unable to eat at the speed of a regular person unless I was wearing headphones and playing some sort of musical accompaniment.

One afternoon, while sitting at a McDonald's around 3 p.m., I forgot to put my headphones on. I noticed that I wasn't chewing more delicately. At the time, I was also researching restaurant reviews to understand the evolution of how we rated restaurants. Suddenly, the answer smacked me right in the face. It was common until the mid-1980s to list the ambient noise levels in restaurants when reviewing them. While some reviewers would just note the noise, some went on to measure it, mostly under the guise of helping a reader decide whether a date there would be quiet and romantic, or loud and happening.

While I had no particular interest in my meals at McDonald's being romantic, it would be very interesting to find out how ambient noise was affecting me and my food intake. As I so often did, I turned to the App Store to help me. There had to be an app for that. Sure enough, I found several applications that were used to measure sound, presumably mostly intended for audio engineers. I downloaded a selection and became utterly bewitched. Every meal I ate turned into an exploration of how my senses were being influenced in ways I was unaware of.

My Filet-O-Fish environment turned out to be 85 to 95 decibels, which is, alarmingly, the equivalent of a blow dryer, leaf blower or even the noise you are subjected to driving a convertible on the highway. Perhaps I was devouring food at far too fast a pace not because of the tempo of my music but because of the assault to my senses. What if McDonald's, as part of their intentional design, wanted the ambient noise levels as high as possible, in order to get me to eat a lot, quickly, then get out of the restaurant as fast as possible? Wait, what if that in-restaurant playground was also put there on purpose, to make noise levels inside even louder? What if those screeching metal chairs, the bathroom doors slamming, those pounding concrete floors, are all intentional design features that McDonald's puts there simply to make the restaurant environment far less pleasant to linger in?

The idea of an engineered noise environment was something I had never considered. But as I ate meals from McDonald's, Subway and Chipotle, I mapped the audio levels for each and every meal. Like so many other data points, what I uncovered changed how I looked at all food environments, not just fast food restaurants.

McDonald's was the cheapest, fastest, saltiest and loudest food you could eat. A normal human conversation is about 60 decibels. McDonald's was consistently at or above 85 decibels— essentially an environment where you can't even talk. And if that's the case, I can guarantee you certainly can't relax.

Even worse, during any meals I ate in front of the television, which happened more than I care to admit, I found that the TV was usually operating at 100 decibels or higher. I was horrified to discover that every situation in which I was consuming food was noisy. (Now picture a picnic on a big grassy knoll overlooking a distant glassy lake. Think about the type of food you tend to consume on a picnic.) Noise matters. A lot.

Were other environmental factors invisibly driving my intake habits as well? What about temperature, humidity, air particulates? The quick list I came up with was exhaustive, so I stuck with some basic environmental factors I could measure easily and log quickly.

I started with light. Light is measured in LUX. A family room in an American home is usually lit to approximately 50 to 70 LUX. Kitchens are brighter—around 110 to 130—and dining rooms come in somewhere between 75 and 85 LUX.

What about McDonald's? You guessed it. McDonald's consistently measured a blinding 200 to 250 LUX. That's as bright as that terrible Walmart lighting, or those office lights that no one will sit still under at a long meeting. Yes, you might be able to see your food, but you also desperately want to escape after about 30 minutes. Fast food restaurants are actually, as it turns out, specifically designed to send you out the door screaming.

Think about the evolution of fast food. Today, we are spending a majority of our food dollars and time on a new breed of restaurant referred to as fast casual. Think Chipotle, Qdoba or Panera. Now consider the differences between traditional fast food and these newer places. Traditional fast food is cheap, fast and unhealthy. Fast casual restaurants are mid-priced, move at a slower pace and tend to have healthier options.

What about the environmental levels at these new spots? McDonald's: bright, hot and loud. Chipotle: dimmer lights, cooler temperatures and quieter kitchens and dining areas. My food intake could be traced not only to the price of the entrée but also to the room it was served in.

HOME IS WHERE THE SENSORS ARE

Think about all the sensors in your home right now, even the ones you don't consider to be "smart." Your thermostat is constantly checking the temperature and making adjustments. Your electric company is monitoring your home energy use and billing you accordingly. The water company knows, down to the ounce, how much water pours through your faucets every day. Smoke detectors are sitting in our ceilings waiting to yell to have their battery replaced, as it takes a lot of energy to sense smoke full time.

These are just simple sensing systems. What about the connected items in our homes? Today many people are adding smart lights, thermostats, plugs, even vacuum cleaners that map out the floors. Both Apple and Google make operating systems for our homes. Google calls theirs Google Home, and Apple's is HomeKit.

Could I extend my surprising discoveries about my eating environments into my home, a place I actually controlled?

Living in my rabbit warren of a basement meant I could consistently hide from the world. But the windows in my bedroom, unlike the windows in my office and den, were not blacked out, because I wanted to be able to enjoy the night air. I have always loved the fall and spring, those wonderful nights you can leave the window open and wake up to birds chirping or leaves rustling outside your window.

I had just hit a patch of rough sleep. Nothing had changed in my carefully orchestrated sleep rituals, but I had started waking up every night just before 3:30 a.m. It was making me feel a little crazy, if for no other reason than it was happening so consistently, and of course, I couldn't get back to sleep. What was waking me up, and could my data help me get back to having a good night of sleep?

My growing interest in the environment had recently led to the purchase of an indoor weather station that I had seen at CyborgCamp. This nifty little machine, called a Netatmo, was small, cylindrical and quite futuristic looking. The idea behind the Netatmo was to learn about things like air quality, temperature, humidity, light and even sound, wherever the station was based. Various apps on my phone were already gathering a lot of this type of information when I was out and about. Now I would be able to better understand the environment in my own home.

My first thought was to put my Netatmo indoor weather station in the kitchen or living room, but what if I could use it instead to learn more about my sleep?

Each life project was turning out to be not one, but two lessons. I learned something new about my life, and I learned about why I wanted to know. So many of the problems in my life were not problems so much as they were opportunities to understand why and how I structured my thinking. Maybe I was being held hostage, not by the issues in my life, but by the way I was thinking about them.

The idea of combining data with my life wasn't new, yet looking at data collecting through the lens of my lifestyle started to take center stage. If I was focused on health, rest, nurturing and recovering, then the tools, applications, sensors and services were selected for that purpose.

Maybe you want to try to sleep better, but after a few apps, podcasts and new skills you decide it's still not enough. By examining your environment, you can take your understanding of sleep to the next level. To that end, I spent a week going to sleep only after manically checking my Netatmo stats, then doing the same after I woke up each morning. Each night, I checked the app to see if conditions were right for sleep. Temperature at 69, humidity around 45 percent and some light music, preferably classical—these were my goals. This little concoction of settings usually did the trick, at least if I hadn't had too crazy a day.

The first few mornings after I woke up with the indoor weather station, I couldn't wait to check out my new data! It was just as exciting as that feeling of looking to see if anyone commented on your last-minute Facebook post before you hit the sack.

Just like my body, it seemed the room did cool slightly through the night. There were also noticeable shifts in air quality, things like changes in humidity and air particulates throughout the day that seemed to stabilize at night. Slowly but surely, as I studied the environment of my sleep lab, I could start to see what made some nights better and some nights worse for sleep.

I began with air quality. I had never really understood the concept before. How was my room air quality changing so much? As it turned out, everything from rambunctious dogs (I had two) to visits from the cleaning lady (overzealous vacuuming) changed the air quality in my home quite drastically. It took me weeks to isolate when these changes would happen and trace them to their source, and then I could make simple changes, like airing out a room with an open window or asking the cleaning woman not to vacuum before a night where sleep was critical.

As I gained greater control over my environment and body, I was able to plan my sleep. For instance, if I knew I was going to be traveling early in the morning, I made sure to get extra rest two days before the trip. I knew it was useless to try to sleep the night before, because I would be too anxious that I might miss my alarm, not to mention that inevitably, in the rush to prepare for a trip, I almost never had gotten enough exercise that day.

If I needed to make a doctor's appointment or get a haircut, I decided which day of the week would be best and how I might sleep the night before as criteria for when to book the appointment. My calendar was no longer open for any type of appointment. My days were data—all filled with things like metrics on nutrition, sleep, activity and mindfulness. Apple now uses all these same characteristics in their Health and Home apps, which blows my mind. Life lived merely as a platform for developers to exploit is a dark future I have long imagined. I just had no idea it would come around quite this quickly.

My fears about a platform-driven life devoid of choice are relatively simple. Let's for a moment take a look at the autonomous nature of our social and dating lives. Apps, developers and corporations mediate many of our relationships.

In the near future, as our health, home and automobile are turned into software platforms, we'll end up locked into applications that we may not need or, worse, that may exploit your vulnerabilities.

I have never worried deeply about the data we give to big companies every day; no, I worry about our ability to understand where our habits come from. The applications we use every day are more than just software programs—they are habits. Within each app you download, you will be conditioned into a few new habits.

A smart home is a giant piece of software where the only options are the ones built into the applications that are used to control it.

In the future, Home Depot will be organized by operating system, not improvement project, and house flippers will just convert one software platform to another.

Who hasn't been burned at home by a software upgrade gone wrong or having to replace an entire system because it's no longer supported?

About two months into my Netatmo experiment, and several weeks into wondering about my early morning wake-ups, I happened upon something key to answering one of my biggest questions in a decade of logging data. While browsing the web, I stumbled across a site that had API connections for both Fitbit and Netatmo.

Many years ago, programmers realized they needed a way to connect the massive systems that we use every day. These connections between behemoth websites and web software are called APIs, or application programming interfaces. APIs make everything we do possible. Without them, the web would just be a series of sites that didn't share information. If you think your password headaches are big now, in a world without APIs you'd spend all your time online reentering information.

APIs are the invisible locks and keys that allow you to share information between the millions of places your data lives, hides and mingles with other data. The data of your life is like a massive escort service, with the APIs in your life like the madam of the house, deciding who gets in and for how long.

Once I figured out how to link my Fitbit data to my Netatmo stats, I logged into both systems and waited for a few seconds as the website merged my data. I would now be able to see my body and my bedroom synced up in one single view. Up until now, most of my guesswork had been, well, guesswork, using some combination of experimentation, observation and the process of elimination.

When the data had finished syncing up, I scrolled through to find my 3:20 a.m. wake-up time. Sure enough, at 3:17 a.m., there had been a change in my room. Although it was only the slightest bit different than normal, the culprit was increased ambient light. I checked the night before, then the night before that. Yes, it seemed as if every night, someone or something between 3:10 and 3:20 a.m. was lighting up my room.

Cars driving by, full moons and other illuminating anomalies happened frequently in my basement, of course, but the regularity of this data blip fascinated me. Perhaps not surprisingly, it also correlated to a marked increase, for just a few seconds, of ambient noise. Maybe I had a ghost? Were my dogs playing poker in the middle of the night?

A serendipitous meeting a few days later would answer my question. I was getting in my car when I saw my neighbor, who I didn't know very well, despite having lived next door to her for ten years. I stuck my head out the window to say hello and ask her how she was doing.

"Oh, I'm so tired. I started working a new shift at the hospital so I'm not getting home until really late these days."

In a flash, my mind raced back, as it so often did, to my data.

"I'm so sorry to hear that. How late are you working?" I asked, perhaps a little too eagerly.

"My shift is over at 2 a.m., but by the time I get out and get home, it's almost 3:30 in the morning some nights."

I had found my answer. That night when I went to bed, I closed the bedroom window that faced my neighbor's driveway, and I carefully pulled some maroon sheet makeshift drapes across my windows, hoping to defend myself against the assault on my environment.

Alas, I still woke up at 3:20 a.m. that night. But when I checked the data in the morning, I found that the Netatmo hadn't recorded any light or noise. Perhaps my hunch was off. Or was it? Perhaps I had just become so accustomed to waking up at that time that I was conditioned at this point. Upon further reflection, I decided to wait it out. Sure enough, after a week, my 3:20 a.m. wake-up slowly but surely started going away, until finally I was back to sleeping happily through the night.

YELLING MY WAY TO PEACE

I wasn't done with my data Jedi training yet. My career was taking off to new levels of success, but one of my greatest challenges at companies was other people.

On my desk in the basement, my warren of technology, right next to my three 23-inch monitors, sat another Netatmo. This one was doing all the same jobs as the Netatmo in my bedroom, capturing light, temperature, air quality, humidity and noise, but I also had something extra at my desk—an alarm of sorts. I knew if I listened to music too loud, I would get distracted when I was trying to be productive. So I created a little program that dimmed my lights if the music in my office rose over 79 decibels. It was my *work, don't party* alert.

One day, while in a fight with my boyfriend, I yelled something loudly, and the lights dimmed a few moments later. I had forgotten about the *don't party* alert. Suddenly the power of my environment over my mood became obvious. What if there were a voice threshold for speaking that showed agitation? If most of the conversations I had were at 65 to 75 decibels, what if I were to create a simple alarm for 76 decibels? I started out by just measuring my normal talking voice using a microphone app on my phone, and I did so again during work conference calls. These calls were a great place to capture sustained prattle from myself and my coworkers without anyone knowing I was data-recording them.

As soon as I had some established baselines, I set up the agitation alarm. Like magic, within days I started to see the fruits of my labor. Conference calls became visible, and the agitation of a group was making my house blink like a disco. No longer was I getting caught off guard—now everything was being alarmed. People started commenting after a few months how calm I seemed lately. My boss told me I was showing greater maturity in dealing with the challenges of our large team. No one knew that each time I was on a call, I had the support of my own voice showing me how to behave, one blink at a time.

In the midst of all my traveling in 2014, Samantha Murphy Kelly, a journalist at CNN, who at the time was with Mashable, the popular online consumer news site, had reached out to me. The day the story was published, I woke and, as usual, went immediately to check my sleep stats on my phone, but before I could even look, I found hundreds of Twitter mentions about the story. I clicked on the link for the article: "Meet the 'Most Connected Man' in the World." In many ways, this was the article that would clarify for me for the first time the depth of what I had been doing for so many years.

When Samantha and her film crew had turned up at my house weeks earlier, I had forgotten to turn off some of the triggers that were monitoring me at that time. During the interview, Samantha had asked me some questions about my mom. I became slightly emotional as I explained the gift she had given me all those years earlier, and what my journey had been like between then and now.

I choked up a bit and slumped over, and my posture belt caught my posture change. My heart rate started to race, and my voice lowered and shook. Suddenly the lights in the room dimmed and slow calming music started to play. Samantha looked at me wide-eyed. The room was clearly responding to my feelings.

She mentioned this in the piece, and although I knew what

I had been doing all this time, for some reason, seeing it in this piece crystallized for me what I had accomplished. I had taken all this data and created feedback loops that had actually changed my perception of myself. Think of it as a tap on the shoulder. Some people get alerts when it's going to rain. I wasn't that different, really. In my house, when a storm's coming in, the lights turn purple and the song "Purple Rain" by Prince begins to play.

You see, anything I could collect, I could create an action for. My smart home wasn't just a house filled with devices, making the need for a full-time remote a reality. I was my own remote control. No buttons required.

Maybe instead of giving our data away so that big corporations can make money off us, we should demand that corporations start taking better care of us, their customers. Home automation could be used for good—for mood management, combating depression and overcoming loneliness. Maybe it's time.

The latest offerings from Apple and Google have no screens at all. Apple's AirPods, the in-ear speaker, and HomePod are examples of the tech giant's latest offerings. You interact with these devices by tapping them or speaking to them directly. The trend of wearing technology *on* our bodies, as we saw with Fitbits and Apple Watches between 2012 and 2014, is slowly being replaced by technology *inside* our bodies, as with AirPods, and *inside* our homes, as with Alexa and HomePod.

The implications of a world where you are immersed in technology at home, in the car, on and in your body, without screens to look at, is transformative in ways the general population can't yet understand. Through my "most connected" status, I have experienced this world and its potential. Next time you worry about your kids or spouse looking at an OLED screen, take a deep breath and remember that the future is coming, and these screens are going away.

Think about how you use software today. You download an application, and you start to arrange your life around it. The screen tells you what you are allowed to do with the app and you find a way to fit those behaviors into your current life. You learn when and how you use the application to book appointments, watch videos or connect with others. You bend your practices around the technology. Applications use people, not the other way around.

Software that is dependent on a screen makes *you* the tool; it's a tough conversation we seem to be unwilling to have, but thankfully it's a temporary problem. Take a step back and consider self-checkout at the grocery store. Most of the time you approach the checkout, start scanning your groceries, pay with a credit card and leave. Upon more profound exploration of our self-checkout experience, it's apparent that we are being manipulated. The self-checkout has a specific order, speed and direction in which you must scan your groceries. You carefully wait to put them into bags, making sure not to hesitate too long and cause the machine to think you're trying to slip that 20-pound turkey into your back pocket.

Self-checkouts are retail dances where the machines metaphorically lead you in a Fred Astaire dance comedy of merchandise bliss! You can see how the evolution of this old style of using technology is evolving by examining the Amazon Go stores opening up in Seattle. In an Amazon Go store, you put the items in your basket and walk out. You don't wait in line to robotically move through a series of screen-prompted steps. In a big-brother style of surveillance, Amazon has installed thousands of cameras and sensors in the store ceiling and on the shelves. The Amazon Go grocery store is an example of how our homes will soon start to function. So let's think about downloading a new *habit* instead of an app.

After several nights of not sleeping well, let's say you decide to download the better sleep habit. (I know Apple is working on this type of sleep function for release in 2019.) The better sleep habit installs on your phone, then connects to your home, car and schedule through a series of permissions that you grant. Slowly the habit service examines your routines and life. First, the service establishes what is normal for you. Where do you sleep and where do you work? What time do you leave for work and what time do you come home? Next, the app understands how much you move during the day and how much time you spend in meetings, stuck in traffic or even standing in line.

Soon your better sleep habit starts to consider the weather and the time of year and compares this against an extensive database of people like you to begin to understand where and when you can start your new habit.

There is no need to look at your phone; your better sleep habit is going to coordinate with all the devices in your life. It gets to work by slowly adjusting the lights in your bedroom several moments before sunrise when you are in your lightest stage of sleep. By understanding your location and watching your sleep from the Apple Watch on your wrist, the new habit slowly brings up the lights to gently awaken you.

Within a few moments, you cover your head and decide to go back to sleep, so your watch starts to vibrate on your wrist, a gentle tapping, not much different from how your mother would wake you up when you were just a small child.

As you jump in the shower, your smart speaker lets you know about the weather, traffic and your appointments for the day and offers to text your first appointment letting them know the traffic is going to be bad and then delays your appointment by 30 minutes.

While stuck in the anticipated traffic, your car looks to the habit to understand if there is anything you might need to help you prepare for the day. In your browse music selections available, you see a podcast on better sleep and eating right. *Funny, how did the car know to offer me that? And it's by one of my favorite podcast hosts!*

Upon arriving at work, you head to back-to-back meetings. Then somewhere near lunchtime, you get a tone in your Air-Pod and you glance down at your watch. The habit is offering to order you lunch, so you don't get too far behind today. With a tap on the watch face, a healthy carb-free lunch is ordered. It's waiting for you in the lobby within 45 minutes.

Near the end of a day that has stretched into its tenth hour, a text message is sent to your spouse letting him know you'll be home late and offering to create a dinner reservation at your favorite restaurant that's walking distance from the office.

You spend 25 minutes walking to dinner to meet your better half and are welcomed with a big hug. The heaviness of another ten-hour day is undeniable, and a bit of empathy goes a long way. On your wrist, you get an alert saying to skip the wine unless you can finish it by 7:30 p.m.! Just enough time, whew. You quickly order wine and throw it back; the alcohol is not going to have a chance to interfere with your sleep. After dinner, you walk back to your car, and by then, the traffic that usually clogs your drive home has cleared.

When you get in bed, your smart speaker offers to play some gentle music, and the lights go from a soft shade of amber to a lavender glow. The room temperature takes on a coolness that invokes the cuddle factor, and the dehumidifier starts to evaporate the day's moisture from your room and home. Near 10:30 p.m., the lights blink once, asking you if you'd like to go to sleep for the night. It doesn't matter. At this point, you're already fast asleep.

In this scenario, there were little to no interactions with screens, and your phone's better sleep habit orchestrated what seemed to be a day perfectly made for good sleep, low stress and connecting to those you love.

This downloadable habit is the reality of the world we live in now, today, as you read this book in 2018, and the scenario above is something I created in 2013, not 2020, though I had to invent the tech myself. Pretty soon, it will be done for us. In the future we will look to health-care providers to send us home with digital prescriptions, downloadable habits we install that slowly upgrade our health.

IOT, the technology that says everything can be smart and connected, is more about a life after screens that helps you interact with the things you value, not your schedule. This is a critically important time in our evolution. We stand at the precipice of a new era of technology and health. Let's hope the tech giants get this one right.

CARS: THE FUTURE OF IOT

One day I saw an ad for Progressive, an auto-insurance company. Flo, their overly vanilla, friendly television spokesperson was saying how I could save money if I just installed their device in my car. Maybe this would help me better understand how I behaved outside my home, when I was in the real world. If that little sensor could save me 15 percent on car insurance, it could probably also act as a body camera for my car. So I got one.

In the name of owning my own data, at least to some extent, I soon ditched the Progressive sensor and purchased an Automatic one. (This company, like many other of the Data Main Street USA vendors over the first half of this decade, has since been acquired by one of the mega content and tech vendors.) The Automatic sensor looked like a little cigarette lighter that plugged into the smart port under my dashboard, then I just had to download an app to my phone to connect it to my car. Now, when I drove, I got real-time feedback on my speed, position, hard braking, sudden accelerations and so on. I even got a cost per trip. (No, don't worry, I did not look while I was driving!)

I was an information-generating machine. One of the first observations I had about my driving data was just how aggressive my driving was. Hard stops and sudden accelerations, two of the data points the sensor collected, were telltale signs of driving a little too hard, and it turns out, they were very indicative of my mood. The sensor didn't just collect my driving information, it provided feedback. As I raced quickly from a light that had just turned green, a subtle beep would sound. When I crossed the speed limit, another alert would go off.

What was behind my hard stops and sudden accelerations? Progressive certainly knew that if I was always racing along, I might be more likely to get into an accident. But Progressive didn't know me. Now that I had access to my own data, I could dig far deeper.

Does the time of day have anything to do with your driving behavior? What about how long you have been driving or sitting in traffic? For me, I found that leaving for appointments with anything less than an hour of buffer time would increase my aggressive driving. Yup, a full hour of leeway was required for me to drive like a civilized human as opposed to a crazed warlord driving his own tank. But leaving too early could also be bad, because if I had too much time to get where I was going, I called, texted and even took photos for my Instagram feed while driving. Too much time to spare, and I became a distracted driver—cue the hard braking.

Other insights fascinated me as well. For example, I drove better when it rained. I also found that I stayed to the speed limit on highways, but not on smaller streets.

A few years after my time with the Automatic sensor, I moved to a different car operating system. In 2015, Apple and Google created operating systems for cars. Just like with each new iPhone, I went to the local VW dealership and didn't ask for a certain color, make or model of car. No, I asked for the line that supported Apple CarPlay. I was aware of the irony that I was about to spend $35,000 on a really fancy iPhone case. But in reality, understanding the data of my car and the systems that would use that data was of vital importance to me.

In 2017, I leased a Tesla, the ultimate piece of connected technology: it drives itself, is always connected to the internet and warns me if I'm driving like a jackass. The Tesla will actually lock you out of features like cruise control or assistive driving if you are driving too aggressively.

Your home, work, school, car and church are all becoming smart, but that doesn't mean you are off the hook on understanding technology. Before you plug in a new lamp, install the latest adapter or wire up the classroom, here are three tips for getting the most out of your environment and protecting your family and life from Amazon, Google and Apple.

First, don't lose your ability to make a choice by limiting your interface. Second, make IOT part of the family. And, finally, avoid devices that take your data and run.

Don't unplug the house.

ENVIRONMENT TIPS

✦ **BEWARE OF LOSING CHOICE:** Smart objects reduce choice—choose them wisely.

✦ **MAKE TECH PART OF THE FAMILY:** Make IOT part of your family's discussions and routines.

✦ **AVOID DATA-HOARDING DEVICES:** Don't buy devices that keep the data to themselves.

BEWARE OF LOSING CHOICE

Smart objects reduce choice—choose them wisely.

We no longer go to the internet, we are the internet. Just as a smartphone isn't very useful without a person tethered to it, the internet is nothing without us.

Over the next decade, our cars, homes and offices will continue to fill with gadgets, buttons and services, all geared toward making our lives easier. But I think we have an opportunity to actually make our lives better.

Next time you go out and buy a smart gadget for your house, and before you have someone throw you the proverbial "You're going to get hacked and your whole family will have to run for their lives and hide as if they are in a remake of *The Purge*" line, take a moment and think about IOT and what this device is going to do for you.

Many of the smart objects we place in our homes don't do much for our health, and that is a grave mistake. Just as DVRs made commercials intolerable and smartphones made waiting for anything avoidable, smart objects like AI are going to take away the last fundamental thing we value as humans: choice.

If you must get a smart speaker, give it only one task: make it an overpriced kitchen timer and no more. If you become dependent on the defaults the speaker offers you, the result will be that you never search for anything more. The reality of a smart speaker is that it is unwilling and incapable of offering you a choice. If you ask a smart speaker for the weather, you get the weather from that speaker's provider. If you ask a smart speaker for music, you get the music that speaker can offer you. You don't get to choose. This is fundamentally important: after the visible internet disappears, which is happening now, the choices in how you experience the internet will be made by others. And those people may not have the time or inclination to consider your particular circumstances.

MAKE TECH PART OF THE FAMILY
Make IOT part of your family's discussions and routines.

The path that AI is blazing through our lives is unavoidable, but it can be on our own terms. While this flies counter to the advice I just gave about limiting your interaction with AI, it is a more realistic method for some. In my family, we make AI part of our meal preparation. We use it for measurement conversions: "Alexa, what's 3 ounces in grams?" We use it for timers: "Alexa, set a timer for 15 minutes." We use it for learning: "Alexa, what's the history of pizza?"

Sometimes I stand in my kitchen and marvel at how connected we are with life after a screen.

AVOID DATA-HOARDING DEVICES
Don't buy devices that keep the data to themselves.

IOT devices have a lot of data, much of which isn't protected but still isn't available to you. Make sure to buy devices that give you access to the data that drives them. If it's a smart-home thermostat, make sure it allows you to see the trends in your home environment. If it's a smart washer or dryer, make sure you can figure out how much water it is using.

When possible, try to look at devices that show you data over time or use other data sources. Devices that integrate with other services will yield greater value in the long run than one-off solutions for sleep or environmental comfort. Many device manufacturers today will give you the devices for what seems like a reasonable price but then charge you to access the data. This trend of charging us for the right to buy back our own data is a growing concern and something that we need a cyborg Ralph Nader for. All the data in the world won't do you much good if you keep giving it away to everyone else and keep nothing for yourself.

PART FIVE

WISDOM
(2014–2016)

Spirituality and Self-Love

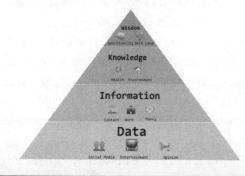

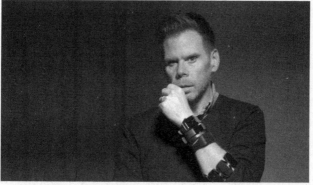

"We don't know how to measure what we care about, so we care about what we measure."

—Richard Tapia

At the start of this journey I promised you digital salvation, and if you've made it this far in the book, you're invested. Let's take your digital salvation one step further by examining the concept of wisdom.

Wisdom is something beyond the data, information and knowledge of technology. In the second decade of the twenty-first century, we need something timeless and more in line with the thinking of Dan Harris, the author of *10% Happier*, the de facto standard in analog spirituality; or Deepak Chopra's enlightened world; or perhaps even a *SuperSoul Sunday* episode you find on Oprah's OWN YouTube channel. We need a new, more modern definition of wisdom.

While it may be a popular opinion to believe we are hopelessly addicted to our technology in a food-sensitive, ADHD, hyper-distracted world, it's not my belief at all. And I hope it won't be yours when we are done. So let's explore technological wisdom, which I define as the ability to remove judgment from your interactions with computing.

That's it. You can close the book now. You're enlightened. Ok, maybe not quite yet. Actually I think it's a lot to ask; removing judgment is a tall order for most people, especially when it comes to technology and our use of it. Judgment is, after all, the key operating principle of technology and humanity. We share that with our mechanical friends—machines just judge more rapidly than we do. What is a computer but a series of 1s and 0s that get turned on and off? Each decision in the blink of an eye, an instantaneous yes or no.

The judgment I'm talking about is what you experience with many people, most of the time, when interacting with today's technology, social systems and devices. Judgment comes spilling out of us so naturally. Spelling mistakes in emails we receive, text messages when someone should be asleep, the Facebook photos of the too perfect vacation shot from the beach or the screenshot of 25,000 steps on your first day off the sofa after a bout of depression.

Technology is breeding a type of cynicism about our fellow humans by rewarding certain behaviors and hiding others. Technology then goes a step further by removing interactions with strangers. There is not a lot of talking in a world of "frictionless" commerce.

If we think that Silicon Valley is coming to fix this mess, we may be disappointed. I can promise you, things are going to get far more difficult before they get easier. So to be technologically wise, we have to focus on ways to decrease our judgment by examining our bias and changing the way we use our technology. This chapter is dedicated to the pursuit of finding the Buddha on your iPad.

In the final part of my journey, I'm going to share the darkest part, where turning myself into a number drove me to the brink of deep depression, isolation and rage. I started where many people do when faced with emotional pain: meditation. It was time to become the world's most connected man, to myself.

11

Spirituality: Technology Isn't Making You a Bad Person

Not All Attention Is Created Equal

BECOMING A MINDFUL CYBORG

Can you attain a deep spiritual awakening using your iPhone? At the end of my journey, I realized: true digital health means treating yourself well.

As I've said, if you open your iPhone and look for the health app, your life gets broken down into four quadrants: activity, nutrition, sleep and mindfulness. It would seem that all you need to be a complete human at the end of the second decade of the twenty-first century is a data plan, a smartphone and a wearable health tracker.

Yet a Fitbit won't make you run, the MyFitnessPal app won't put better food in your mouth and a Beddit sensor can't keep you from staying up past bedtime. Likewise, your Headspace or Simple Habit app can't create a mindfulness practice and force you to use it.

Using technology for spiritual practices goes against everything we teach in today's culture. The one set of people whose advice we might take seriously in becoming more mindful, the Buddhists, advocate in fact for a world where technology is completely abandoned. The traditional spaces of worship in our society are entirely free of technology. If you ever have the chance to visit a meditation retreat, you'll quickly discover that all books, pens, paper and even clocks are carefully hidden away in these spaces.

But I am advocating the need for a deep spiritual practice that includes technology. Spirituality has played some small part in every piece of technology innovation over the past 500 years: The first books ever printed on a movable-type press were Bibles. Within years of the advent of radio and TV, we had televangelism being piped into our living rooms. And no sooner was the first web page put up than there were chat groups for Christians. Yet today, when we think of technology and spirituality, too often we focus on radical fringe religious groups: transhumanists, bio-hackers and Singularitarians (followers of the Ray Kurzweil ideology that computers and AI will and should wake up).

We all know that we desperately need to address the realities of technology's place in our culture right now. We need to look at what I call the rise of the mindful cyborg and talk openly and frankly about the fear, uncertainty and doubt that we all share in our technology-rich world.

There are times that I feel deep shame when I pick up my phone to log a meal, check the weather or see my next appointment. And I know for certain that these feelings of shame are the exact opposite of the feelings of gratitude that come with a deep faith or spiritual practice. Yet here we are, sitting in coffee shops, spying on our family, checking our lack of steps and logging the 50 grams of sugar in our spiced pumpkin hot chocolate. How did we get here, how do we get out and how does technology play a role in that journey?

The basics of a spiritual practice using technology are available to us as of the writing of this book. All the large wearable technology companies have included mindfulness as part of their technology. A few times a day, your Apple Watch will tell you to breathe deeply and exhale as a rhythmic icon slowly pulsates on your wrist. That mindful moment you just experienced with your watch will then get logged in your Apple Health app.

If you've ever downloaded a meditation app, I'm sure you've been asked to sit in a comfortable position with your hands resting in your lap and start focusing on your breath. But it's not just in our everyday technology that we find mindfulness. If you travel to some parts of the southern United States, right after the Chick-fil-A and Fox News apps, you'll see a variety of different Bibles in the top 10 list.

Spirituality is part of our technological journey whether we like it or not, and these are just the obvious spiritual tools for people seeking a little extra redemption through their phones. But there are so many other outlets for the deeper good in the universe if you look closely at our technology consumption. Viral videos of someone doing something good, Facebook disaster check-ins to help find missing loved ones or the onslaught of patrons for GoFundMe campaigns have become today's digital churches, where we band together to help the people in our communities through life's toughest battles.

As a practicing mindful cyborg, I have tried a lot of different techniques to bring some humanity into my technology, whether it was using an EEG headband like Muse to train my brain to be aware of certain brain-wave patterns or just simply sitting with my Buddhify app. I feel like there isn't anything I wouldn't at least try to hack my spiritual side.

INSTALL CHRIS 1.0

My search for meaning, *my* meaning anyway, began in child-hood. I was obsessed with card catalogs and libraries, and the potential I sensed within them. My mother's aunt would often take my brother and me to her church on Sundays. There I wit-nessed people filled with the spirit, and I studied the customs and rituals of the evenly seated rows of parishioners, all wor-shiping not a room full of books, but a single book, the "truth." Some of my friends would be fearful of the occasional trip to church, but I found the ordered nature of time and space, along with the rituals around communication and sacrifice, to be right up my alley.

Fast-forward to my freshman year of high school, when I started finding my salvation in bookstores. What was it about the self-help section that both inspired and shamed me? For starters, long before I understood the societal view of people who were "seeking" help, I noticed that this was where books on self-discovery were kept.

Inside the Little Professor bookstore at the Carrollton mall in Maryland, near the back wall, just past the bathroom, there was a row of shelves unlike others in the store. The books here took on widely different sizes, colors and shapes. Their titles were embossed onto glossy, bright, eye-catching covers: *Co-dependent No More*, *Zen and the Art of Motorcycle Maintenance*, *Creative Visualization*.

Even today I can close my eyes and see the shelves of titles in front of me, and a profound sense of relief still washes over me, that all of these books, and the wisdom they contained, would be able to finally answer those questions I couldn't stop asking: Who are you? Why are you here? Whose hands are these?

But why were these books hidden in the back of the store?

And why didn't I see other teenagers in this area? Maybe there was something wrong with me? My very first purchase during my freshman year of high school was *The Road Less Traveled* by M. Scott Peck. I opened the first page of that book, and with blinding clarity, I remember reading the very first sentence: "Life is difficult." *My God, this guy gets me*, I thought. *He understands my problems.* When I got home, I hid the book under my mattress. My quest for wisdom had started, and it wasn't going to get easier from here.

✦ ✦ ✦

Panic attacks are something I have dealt with my entire life, and during high school, one of my episodes got so scary, I thought I was going to die. I walked down the hall and pushed my parents' door open. "Dad, there's something wrong with me."

"What's wrong Christopher?"

But I didn't know how to put what I was feeling into words.

"I think I'm dying. My chest is really hurting and my heart is beating so fast."

With a voice that was from another time, and a tone that felt like he had been waiting my entire life to share this piece of wisdom, my dad replied: "It's just life, Christopher. It's hard sometimes, but you'll be fine." I went back to bed with questions echoing in my head that would never truly be answered. *Why* was life so hard? Would I be fine?

The boy who had so many philosophical questions was replaced by a guy who filled his life with technology. The philosopher was dead, long live the technologist. Screens could say anything, though they lacked the permanence of books and ideas older than the bookstores in which I found them.

Many years later, I was sitting in my psychiatrist's office, talking about how often I had panic attacks, when Dr. Lewis

started asking me about my childhood. Dr. Lewis special-
ized in acceptance and commitment therapy (ACT). I often
referred to her in the early days as a reformed pill pusher who
had found Buddhism.

In essence, ACT helps people come to terms with their
lives as they are and stop resisting their thoughts. ACT doctors
aren't anti-drug as much as they believe in a motto of "skills
over pills." For me, pills over skills had always been more efficient, but since, back then, I weighed 320 pounds, was smoking two packs of cigarettes a day and had a raging drug and
junk-food habit, I was willing to admit my solutions weren't
working. I badly needed to find a better solution, and my medical doctor was only willing to write me prescriptions for blood-
pressure medication and give me some pointed lectures about
learning to eat better.

My work with Dr. Lewis would mark the beginning of my
focus on spirituality and wisdom. I spent long days and countless hours rehearsing what I would say to her, but more importantly, also repeating what she said to me. This active
retraining of my thoughts started to transform my brain, and
I slowly managed to wean myself off the cocktail of benzodiazepines, antidepressants and assorted drugs that I had been
on for so many years.

I learned from Dr. Lewis that it was ok to be sensitive, that
my panic attacks, dissociation and even depression served a vital purpose to protect me from distressing situations or
people. This acceptance would soon lead me to a group of practicing Buddhists in Boulder and then eventually to a meditation group in Nashville.

I had spent so much time amassing data, gleaning information from that data and attempting to turn it into knowledge that, yes, I had become slightly healthier, but I was no

happier. It was time to reach for the highest tier. I needed wisdom.

In my quest for wisdom, I would explore my mental health challenges, including my anxiety and depression, and examine my spirituality and what it meant for me, especially in the face of my technology-driven life. I also resolved to find love, even if that meant learning to be ok alone.

DELETE CHRIS 1.0

In 2014, I was the cover boy for what you could do with a Fitbit, but my still unhealthy body was not going to let me off the hook so easily. I was truly about to hit bottom with my physical and emotional health.

It was early June 2014 in Denver and the weather was glorious. No humidity, beautiful clear skies, so I decided to ride my bike to the mall. The ride would be the furthest I had ever traveled by bike, nearly 12 miles each way, and while it was mostly flat, there were some good hills along the way. I wanted to prove to myself that I was truly getting healthier. At this point, I weighed about 220 pounds, and although I had been consistently working out and eating right for many months now, I was still not ready for the cover of *Men's Health*.

The ride was exhilarating. But it wasn't easy—in fact, it was brutal. All the travel, the stress and the changes in my work life were catching up with me, and despite my months of work to get healthier, I barely made it home. As some sort of odd reward for surviving the trip, I decided I deserved a cigarette. I lit up, feeling hopeless and furious, mad at myself for being in such poor shape, embarrassed about how difficult the trip was for me and stressed about the decisions I would soon need to make about my future.

Panic shot through my body and I felt my heart jump out

of my chest. Another panic attack. I gasped and put out the cigarette as if I had been caught by a preacher or parent. I was having a heart attack, I was sure of it. (Years later I would learn about catastrophizing and how to cope better with these self-narrated negative stories, but for now, I had no coping techniques.)

I was going to die. I had a friend drive me to the hospital. Soon, I was lying on a hospital bed, with IVs hooked up to my arm and EKG leads snaking out of my surgical gown, the screaming machine next to me vibrating with beeps and buzzes, collecting my body's complete meltdown. The irony was not lost on me.

After my blood results came back and my EKG was reviewed, I was cleared. I was not having a heart attack. Slowly over the next two hours, my heart rate returned to normal and I was released. They told me not to smoke and to take it easy bike riding. It turned out that my body was still in control of my life, even if I was in control of my body's data.

In the coming weeks, I forced myself to see a cardiologist to assuage my fears about an imminent heart attack. A battery of tests, monitors and three visits later, Dr. Rougas started asking me about my life. I explained to him in some detail what I had been doing since 2008 and how it had changed me. He gave me a bemused look.

"So all this is good for you?"

I was taken back, astounded that he couldn't see how much good had come from my data project. Then I paused and started to laugh. I guess he had a point. What was the purpose of using technology if it was going to stress you out so much that you didn't know the difference between needing 20,000 steps and needing rest? I had gotten to the point where I was living for a number.

"Listen, you know how to take care of yourself. Why don't

you take some time off and just relax?" Dr. Rougas said. "You're healthy, and your heart is healthy. You're just stressed out."

I left his office feeling calm for the first time in weeks, if not months. When I got home, there was a FedEx envelope on my doorstep. It was from the Healthways executives who had been in the audience back when I presented for the Clinton Foundation. They were offering me a huge salary and a relocation package to Nashville to come work for them full time. Finally, an opportunity to vacate the life that had created so much madness. Did I have the courage to take it?

I wasn't sure. Was I really going to leave my life in Denver behind and start a full-time job in a brand-new place? Yes. I knew it was time to move on.

MOOD PANDA

All the pounds and steps and calorie counts were still automatically being fed into my computer, but after my moment of clarity with Dr. Rougas, I knew that I needed to dig deeper than the numbers; it was time to look at my feelings. But understanding my moods better was a little more difficult than collecting hard data.

I downloaded Mood Panda, an app that helps you log your mood. My first days with Mood Panda were somewhat frightening. The idea of opening an app to share my innermost feelings seemed odd, even to me, yet there was something comforting about seeing the trends in my mood after only a few days. I was, perhaps not surprisingly, all over the map. The only thing I knew for sure was that my mood would be key to deciphering my spirituality.

Some people wear their heart on their sleeve, and I was one of them, so actually sharing my feelings has never been a problem. But logging moods, unlike logging steps, sleep, food and work completed, takes a level of commitment that most people don't fully understand. Still, if you commit to the process, it allows you to very quickly create a map of emotions and to interact with them in a deep and intense way.

Long before you have the strength to meditate for five minutes, you need to start to understand and work with your feelings. I know, even just the phrase "working with your feelings" sounds like one of those awful touchy-feely subjects we hear about during high school assemblies, or from the overly exuberant motivational speakers at required work conferences. But in reality, just working with your emotions in your own way is the fastest approach to understanding what you value and what you don't. Long before we looked to the web for validation of our beliefs, we actually looked inward to understand those beliefs.

Mood-logging can be as easy as keeping a feelings diary or as elaborate as writing down your every waking whim and emotion. But start off slowly. Just jotting down your feelings in a note on your phone is enough.

My ability to keep up a steady, regular written diary has always been on par with my relationship with God. When I needed it, I reached out, but consistency was clearly lacking.

Today there are so many services to help you journal and keep track of your life. I mean, what is Facebook but a public diary of the version of yourself you wish to leave behind? And even Facebook now asks you to add how you're feeling when you post.

Unfortunately, all this does is force the algorithm to send critical updates about your mood to your friends. Back in the 90s, outside my work cube, I hung a small sign that showed 20 different hand-drawn faces, each expressing a different emotion. There was a small frame you could move around the sign to choose which particular one you felt like at any given moment. I tended to use this as a warning to people, but trust me, if you're one of the people who has a feelings sign outside your office, everyone already knows you're a basket case.

YOU IGNORE YOUR FEELINGS WHEN YOU'RE FINE

The first lesson I learned from mood-logging was just how complicated my relationship with myself was. There was a specific logic to my feelings and my ability to log or collect them. If life was going well, and I was happy, I rarely wanted to bother to stop being happy for a second to log those feelings. But if I was feeling fearful, I was far more willing to collect my feelings. It was easy to pull out my phone to log feelings when I was feeling dark or angry. But, oddly, I had no particular desire to log my feelings when I was depressed or anxious.

Have you ever noticed that moments of rage come from seemingly nowhere or how that twinge of anxiety shows up right when everything seems, well, perfect?

My search revealed that these feelings weren't as instant as they appeared, and had I taken time to notice them when my life seemed perfectly fine on autopilot, I could have probably avoided some nasty falls.

When logging emotions, I needed to be diligent so that I could look backward and consider the conditions that led up to these pivots of the heart.

Hours or days before depression, I spend more time online; weeks before anxiety or rage, my music selections slowly change or get reduced.

Our feelings take a long time to manifest, and our ability to understand and decipher them can only be seen in hindsight. The antidote is reprogramming your future, but we'll cover that in depth later.

To that end, as days became weeks and weeks became months, I started noticing patterns. My Mood Panda graph was filling up, and I could see a full spectrum of highs and lows in my life. My moods seemed to mostly stick to a relatively regular cycle except when they didn't. On those days, my bad mood was always attributed to travel, a depressing anniversary of some sort or a deadline.

Once I got the hang of logging my feelings, I was able to use one of my secret Twitter accounts, @dancymood, to correlate my mood with other events. Was I more angry during the week? Did more sleep make me happier? What does how I'm eating have to do with how I'm feeling?

It doesn't take a mood-logging genius to figure a lot of this stuff out, but some conclusions were more obvious than others.

MEANING WELL IS NOT WELL MEANING

My anger, I found, was pretty predictable. If I had periods of inactivity—such as limited computer usage or waiting on hold on the phone or in line—my mood sharpened, and not in a good way. I became hyper-vigilant and protective of my time.

Respect for the order of time is a real trigger for me. The anxiety of waiting, of not getting things done, can be paralyzing. Anger for me always comes at times when I have put myself up against a deadline or I have to deal with someone else on a deadline. Just as some people learn to be one with their breath, for me, watching time tick by in my head is a trigger for anger.

Anger is one of those emotions that we really need more practice with. I've often found that my empathy and compassion are only as deep as my controlled rage. Joking with friends, I know that I've said, with barely hidden aggressiveness, "Don't worry, I'll take care of this, I mean well" with a sinister smirk. My good deeds seem to be undone by my bad attitude more often than I care to admit. On the flip side, I have also found that my levels of anger and rage are often matched by periods of deep reflection. So if I'm honest about measuring anger, it should also always be combined with an active review of how much "good" I thought I was doing. Without fail, the level of my perceived kindness is only matched by the heights of my rage for situations.

If you have trouble with anger, try to do some good deeds for a bit, or just be careful when you help out a friend.

TRAVEL WILL WRECK YOU

Anger was also closely associated with travel. If I was coming or going to some place I didn't normally travel to, such as on work trips, I would always have increased outbursts of anger prior to and during these stressful trips. Not to point out the obvious, but if you've ever stood in line at the airport for a late flight or had a tight connection, I think you understand how anger and travel go hand in hand.

I decided to address anger as my first emotional life hack. I had already life-hacked my diet, sleep and activity. Why couldn't I actively affect my moods?

Once I understood the types of events that triggered me (a term that has so much more cachet in today's climate of micro-aggressions and public freak-outs), I was able to become pro-actively aware of looming meltdowns and figure out ways to work around them.

Getting to the airport three hours early helped. Booking reserved seating helped. Making sure I had the phone number or contact information for the different points of support during my trip helped. I also found that choosing *not* to travel with loved ones could be helpful. Sometimes booking a separate flight and meeting up with each other once that first overly stressful part of the vacation is finished is an easy way to start vacation off on the right foot.

Not surprisingly, the relatively simple act of planning ahead, as well as getting adequate rest and adjusting my schedule

before I arrived, usually did the trick. My angry outbursts
started to decrease.

CHOOSING TO PUT MYSELF IN HARM'S WAY

The next hacking goal required me to practice coping with intense pressure. I wanted to practice resilience well before I
needed it. With the help of my therapist, Dr. Lewis, who was
still overseeing my 20-year withdrawal from antidepressants
and benzos, I started doing something I called the "Loving
Kindness Fight Club." Loving kindness is a Buddhist principle of giving and receiving love for yourself and those near to
you while continuing to focus on even those people who bring
you pain or discomfort.

My goal was to try to inoculate myself against anger by
exposing myself to it on purpose. If ambitious Nobel laure-
ates could expose themselves to radiation to study its effects,
then I surely could force myself to absorb the anger of a stranger
and manage mine in response, right?

The experiments started out rather simply. I would wait
until a big rain- or snowstorm was coming, and I would head
out to the grocery store at rush hour. This is not a joke. I did
this on purpose. I knew this hit all my triggers: waiting in line,
feeling rushed, being surrounded by angry people. It sounds
insane, I know, but for me, it was the best way to learn to feel
anger and accept it.

The first few times nothing happened. People drove horri-
bly, the lines at the store were terrible and people were pushing
and making a scene, yet somehow I just wasn't that angry.

When I went back and looked at my mood data, the problem was pretty obvious. There was no deadline or appointment
that was weighing on me. Yes, people around me were having bad days but they weren't bothering me. The key to my
lack of rage was as simple as not being in a rush. I needed to

manufacture a sense of urgency so I could start to experience authentic pressure. No problem, all my conference calls were now scheduled at the worst possible time—early in the morning, in the middle of rush-hour traffic, several hours after a meal.

Manufacturing the conditions for rage were leading to more insights about anger.

For better or worse, my first attempt at my local Kroger supermarket was a smashing success! I waited until just before a scheduled product release conference call with senior management, then I grabbed my keys and headed out in a heavy storm and drove right to the store. The noise from the parking lot and the crowds made hearing the call difficult and caused my manager to ask, "Where are you? Chris can you put your phone on mute?"

My employer's pleas to control my environment only made me more anxious and angry. All around me, people were coming into the store covered in water, shaking their wet umbrellas all over me and making all sorts of noise. Anger was building. I had done it! For a second, I felt like the Incredible Hulk who was stuck in some middle state, not totally green and shirtless but not a well-kept Bruce Banner either. I stood in the store, saw and felt all my rage and started writing down everything that was happening as if I were an anger scientist.

I observed my voice, my elevated heart rate, the sweat on my lower back, my walking pace, how I chewed my lip, how I glared at people who passed me by, unaware of my tense situation: trying to keep my employer happy with my work while simultaneously trying to shop for more difficult feelings.

Yeah, this is next-level crazy, but when do we get the chance to practice being angry?

WATCHING ANGER ARRIVE

My anger clearly stemmed from my need to control the narrative, either in my environment or in my communication. Have you ever been in an argument with someone where all you can think about is the desire for that person, for just a second, to understand your version of reality? This is critical, because once I realized I wanted validation for my version of an experience, I could start to use this as a sign that I was, in fact, on my way to rageville.

Next the physical signs of anger showed up: respiration, heart rate, walking speed, voice level—all these things changed once I was angry. My voice didn't rise until I started speaking faster—I learned this from putting a sound sensor in my office during phone calls.

Now that I had cracked the code of when anger happened, not only did I start planning everything more carefully but I got serious about my feelings and why I was having them. No longer did I just accept my thoughts as reality; I had to question them, even the happy ones. My six-month journey of exposing myself to toxic people and conditions so that I could learn to have those emotions and isolate them changed me profoundly.

Today I still practice this, but I've downgraded my weapons. Now I use videos, emojis and memes to navigate my feelings. It's a lot easier to blow off steam using the 💩 or a Picard meme than it is to get something off your chest by blowing up at the person making you furious. More about dealing with difficult feelings later!

RECOGNIZING THAT UNFAMILIAR FEELING: IS THIS HAPPINESS?

After I understood the source of my anger, I practiced with happiness. The first thing I needed to clear up was the difference between being happy and feeling content. For my entire life, I thought I wanted to be happy, but what I actually wanted was contentment.

Happy is pretty easy to track. Even strangers know when you're happy. Logging happy is a bit more difficult because no one wants to take the time to check off "completed happiness" on their daily to-do list. Happy is something we just expect to happen, not something we deserve. Culturally, we kind of make a big deal about happy, we define it, photograph it and celebrate it.

Yet if you look at technology, it's really hard to tell if someone is happy. If your friend has gone missing online, maybe they met someone and actually got a life. Have you ever had a friend who suddenly started posting a lot of motivational quotes? If you're like me, the first thing you'll do is wonder if they are ok. There must be something wrong if they have decided to become a one-man Dr. Phil on Pinterest. Surely no one is that happy?

My exploration of happy led me to some deep learning about what I wanted in life. I wanted rest. I wanted good food. I wanted to help other people. I wanted a mixture of a social life and a hermit existence. I wanted people to respect me. I wanted to respect myself.

The challenge of being happy in the digital world is pretty straightforward. I needed to learn how to use my technology to help me understand how to measure the things that I valued. Do you value journaling every day and making at least one meal at home per week? Good, don't track anything but those two things, and measure everything about those two things! Do you value exercise? Well, the challenge again with this goal is the measurement. You value moving, but you don't value 10,000 steps. You get fit by taking steps, not counting them.

What you'll find as you start to move from looking for

happiness to committing to finding your values is that *happy* will take care of itself. You'll end up creating a type of gratefulness toward yourself. By measuring what you value instead of valuing what you measure, you will find happiness.

FROM HAPPY TO GRATEFUL

When I combined practicing gratitude and directing it at others, things started to change. Back when I was working on improving my sleep, I found that there was one type of meditation that really helped me. It wasn't the traditional watch-your-breath Samatha meditation or the chant-based Metta meditation. It was something called gratitude meditation, and when I discovered it, it helped me start to see more profound changes in my spiritual life.

I felt different immediately. Someone would have a meltdown in front of me, and instead of melting down myself, I took notice of my inner dialogue. I would switch my focus to concentrating on being grateful that I was getting another chance to practice getting yelled at.

While these early days of logging feelings, defining what it was that I cared about and figuring out how to communicate it were immature at best, they would lead to profound changes in my life. My journaling actually started to inoculate me against the dark emotions of anxiety and depression.

As I was about to enter this new period of my life with a healthy body, new home and exciting job, I knew I would need these skills. In the list of life stressors, career changes, moving to a new place, the loss of a loved one and physical or mental challenges are all in the top ten. I was doing all top ten at once.

While there was no instant fix that helped me find peace of mind, there are a few changes you can make right away. But first, don't unplug.

SPIRITUALITY TIPS

✧ **LOWER DISTRACTION:** Five things you can change on
your phone right now to take back control.

✧ **THE ART OF APPYNESS:** How to organize apps by
feeling to regain control over your attention.

✧ **WAKE UP TO THIS MOMENT WITH AN ALARM:** Use
alarms, tasks and your calendar to be more present.

✧ **NAME YOUR DEVICES AFTER YOUR VALUES:** Use names
for all of your devices to remind you of what you value
and cherish.

✧ **CONSIDER ALL TECHNOLGY AS A TIME MACHINE:** Learn
to use your technology as if you're in the future and
reprogram your today.

LOWER DISTRACTION

Five things you can change on your phone right now to take back
control.

There are subtle things you can do to push yourself to interact
differently with your tech. For example, are you one of the millions of people who suffer from feeling lost without your
phone, something called nomophobia? Then I want to help you
start to reshape your relationship with your phone.

According to my friend Amber Case, our phones have
become a remote control for reality and, just like a remote
control, they dominate our feelings and environments. Somehow we have gone from casually checking our phone for the
time to obsessively checking our phone for our battery percentage. The amount of energy left in our phone is now
symbolic of the time left in our day, Sunsets and sunrises

have been replaced by the 100 percent and 0 percent of our phone battery label.

Here are five things you can do right now to start to slow down your relationship with your phone:

1. Remove any label that shows you how much battery you have left. Often the dwindling battery percentage on our phone only adds anxiety to our day.

2. Consider changing the time format on your phone to a 24-hour time. If you're in Europe, change the time to 12-hour time. By giving yourself something to think about when you look at the time, you are forced to slow down a bit and confront your out-of-control schedule.

3. Create a completely clear home screen. When you unlock your phone, let the first thing your eyes see be the open expanse of a screen completely free of updates, apps, folders or information widgets.

4. Organize the apps on your phone by icon color. Try it! Instead of placing all the applications on your phone in order of how often you use them, line them up on the screen like a continuous rainbow. When you search for applications by color, you'll start to see your phone as an extension of your mood.

5. Use a different lock screen and wallpaper. Consider placing two images that complement each other on your phone to walk you through the process of unlocking your phone. I've used the moon and the Earth. Day and night. One pet and the second pet. The idea is to allow our minds a way to interact with our phones that broadens our depth of feelings, rather than ignoring them.

THE ART OF APPYNESS

How to organize apps by feeling to regain control over your
attention.

We've all been there, that moment when we are shoulder-surfing someone next to us at the grocery store, looking at the apps they are using or the text message they are composing. I have been known to ask strangers, "What are you using there?" Or I'll ask to see people's phones, after ample assurance that I won't go full-on stalker mode. What makes how people interact with their devices so interesting? Why are we so fascinated with the tools that shape everyone else's life?

Let's explore more ways you can start to organize and use your phone now that you have some of the visual triggers out of the way. You did turn off that battery percentage already, right?

I'll tell you something about myself: I can't have Reese's Peanut Butter Cups in my house. Seriously, I can't. Sometime between the ages of 35 and 50, I lost the ability to control myself when I see them. Quickly I find myself five empty packages deep, feeling sick to my stomach, with a mouth covered in chocolate. The day after Halloween at Walgreens is too much for me to even think about because of the cheap chocolate factor. Well guess what? My phone and specific applications on it are no different. So let's look at some healthy strategies to work through these digital urges.

First, put applications you use too often someplace out of reach. Don't make them easy to get to. Place them up and to the left if you're right-handed or get daring and move all your favorite apps to the second or third screen on your phone. It's just like placing the forbidden candy on a high shelf in your kitchen.

Next, fill your home screen with the apps you don't use

that much, but you want to start using. It's like placing your running shoes next to the front door before going to bed. Again, this forces you to think about what you could be doing, not what you want to do. Use your phone to stretch your mind. Do you find yourself continually spending too much time on Facebook or social media? Delete the apps, turn off the notifications and force yourself to use your browser when you need your fix.

Of course, this doesn't address the root problem of our social media or app habits. The root problem has become the blurred line between our applications and our feelings. So let's treat our apps like feelings and label them as such. For so many people today, it's hard to define our emotions; they are mixed up and recycled with a million other organic reactions competing for a little attention in our overly stimulated brains.

Here's a dare for you, the reader who is considering digital salvation: organize your applications by feelings. Of course, we can't have digital salvation unless we first define what digital sin is. To that end, if you are ever lucky enough to get ahold of my phone, the first thing you'll notice is that a majority of my applications are in folders labeled by sin. Good old-fashioned cardinal sins.

Ask any devoted Christian or Brad Pitt movie buff, and they can probably list the traditional seven deadly sins, which instantly invoke feelings within us. In no particular order, the seven deadly sins are pride, greed, lust, envy, gluttony, wrath and sloth.

On my phone you'll see folders labeled with sins, and inside each folder you'll find the corresponding applications. For example, in my envy folder you'll find banking, invoicing and credit card applications. When I use these applications—reviewing my wealth or dwindling bank balances—I'm reminded of the true nature of my inquiry.

The greed label adorns the folder for applications that are used in my home and car, all the nifty cool geeky gadgets that power my physical life. The greed label is a constant reminder that the real value of physical items is often rooted in coveting them.

No set of downloadable sins would be complete without pride. Pride, the father of all the sins, holds venerable applications like Facebook, Twitter, LinkedIn and Snapchat: all the places I go to get affirmation that I'm doing well, that I am who I think I am.

Don't let this process get you down though! Make sure you create folders for the things you value. I also have folders called "Stillness" and "Kindness." They contain applications for the weather and location-based information like maps and hiking paths.

Are you feeling uncomfortable yet? Good because we are just getting started with your baptism in the digital waters!

WAKE UP TO THIS MOMENT WITH AN ALARM
Use alarms, tasks and your calendar to be more present.

In 2015, I was talking on the phone with a lifelong friend we will call "Kay." I could hear buzzing and beeping in the background. Kay's Apple Watch was vibrating against her wrist, her laptop was digitally pleading with her to pay attention, and finally her phone began shaking violently on the table near her. "Chris, I have to go." The phone call abruptly ended.

The next time I saw Kay, I asked her about that day and what happened. "Oh, I sometimes lose track of time, and I use my phone to remind me of where to be."

Another time, while at the mall with her, I noticed one of her phone alarms go off. "Oh, shit," she exclaimed, "We have to leave, it's time to pick up Jack." Jack is her son, and he attends a special school for autism.

I suspected that she was onto something. "Hey, can you show me how you use your alarms?" I asked.

Kay handed me her phone and I opened the alarm application. Nearly 50 different alarms filled the screens over six pages. These alarms were labeled "Get Jack off to school," "Leave for work," "First period ends," "Check on this" and "Go Home." Where some people may use their alarm function on their smartphone to wake up in the morning, Kay had created an elaborate series of reminders that filled every waking hour of her day.

I'm no stranger to lists and organization—you're reading a book about how I managed the thousands of connections in my life, but I thought that what Kay was doing was some next-level stuff. I started asking people if I could see their alarms. I asked friends, peers and even strangers at conferences. Slowly I discovered that many people were living life dictated by tens, sometimes hundreds, of these audible signals.

In our digital lives, there are three types of software that dictate our time: alarms, reminders and appointments. Appointments are the promise to do something at a specific time and place, yet in an age where it's far easier to cancel a commitment than to order an Uber, appointments have become kind of old-fashioned, the time equivalent of voicemail.

Next, we have reminders, or tasks. I love tasks! Tasks speak to a promise, a specific non-event that you want to accomplish. Tasks are often items we need to complete to make an appointment or event more successful. For some of my friends, tasks have become more like goals.

Finally, it seems as if we have embraced alarms as a culture. Strangely enough, there is nothing flexible about alarms. They lack the preparation of an appointment or the clarity of tasks and instead force all your attention to focus only on a weaponized "now."

I wanted to explore how to make alarms more aligned with my values and less with my time. What if instead of scheduling these jarring screeching alerts to remind you to leave for the airport on time, you set alerts to remind you to "Move slow" or "Focus on what you can control"? These powerful alarms are, in essence, do-nothing alarms, or as we say in Buddhism, "Don't just do something, *sit there!*"

I have set hundreds of these do-nothing alarms over the years on my journey to becoming a mindful cyborg. I even employ emojis in the alarm titles to force my mind to truly take notice of the action. My "Move slow" alarm comes with a charming little turtle peeking out at me. Sometimes I create a random alarm that repeats once a month to remind me of something I want myself to remember, such as, "These are the good times." My alarms act as emotional bookmarks for the browser of my life. It is so easy to turn your alarms from tyrannical life-interrupters to peaceful reminders for your soul.

Alarms are good reminders of mindfulness now, but what can you create for the future? Our phones also have the ability to create reminders or task lists. Reminders function like alarms but in the forms of lists: a list for the grocery store or a packing list for a vacation. Reminders are powerful in a way that alarms are not, as they can be set up for locations. Put this book down, pick up your iPhone or Android and whisper: "Hey Siri / Ok Google, remind me to smile at the cashier when I get to Whole Foods." Next time you get to the grocery store, your phone will tell you to smile at the cashier.

At first, creating a breadcrumb trail to encourage behaviors in your future self might seem a little odd. But remember, you are reprogramming yourself. In a world short on wisdom and overflowing with data, remembering to smile at an underpaid cashier will do more for your soul than hours at a gym.

Chicken soup for the cyborg soul is a real thing. You are starting to practice it here, now.

NAME YOUR DEVICES AFTER YOUR VALUES

Use names for all your devices to remind you of what you value and cherish.

We've all been to that friend's house with the Wi-Fi name that is silly, "Too Fly for a Wi-Fi," or "Pay for Your Own Damn Wi-Fi." Wi-Fi names are this generation's bumper stickers, and they always give people who join them a chuckle. Yet our devices join more than Wi-Fi networks. We join Bluetooth speakers, headphones, watches, home systems, cars and each other via file transfers like AirDrop.

Think about it, every device you have in your life has a name, and you probably spend a good amount of time joining these other machines in a tiny network of you. I often refer to this as the "Inner-net" as opposed to the internet that we are all used to. Inside this network of you, you're reminded constantly of the devices you are sharing information with.

Shouldn't all this connectedness be a reminder to you about what you value? Couldn't all these connections also be a reminder to someone else? When people visit my home and join the Wi-Fi, they join "Be Kind to Yourself." My watch, laptop and earphones are named, respectively, "Compassion," "Open Your Heart" and "Listen to Your Body." Whenever I connect, share files or change devices, multiple times throughout the day, I get reminders to listen to my heart. When I use my phone as a hotspot, I get asked by my laptop, "Do you wish to join Open Your Heart?" And of course, the answer is yes.

The world's great spiritual leaders would surely have had no problem with technology designed like this. And hey, if you're a traveling Jehovah's Witness or Latter-day Saint, this

is a pretty cool way to spread the message while surfing You-
Tube.

CONSIDER ALL TECHNOLGY AS A TIME MACHINE

Learn to use your technology as if you're in the future and
reprogram your today.

If there were a universally understood definition of transcen-
dence, enlightenment or a higher spiritual plane, it would be
a feeling of timelessness. All technology acts as a time machine.
If our day seems fast or our dread seems slow, more often
than not the technology in our lives is enriching that experience. As we think about using technology to make ourselves
happier, we need to look closely at the messages technology is
sending us. This chapter has been about reprogramming your
now and your *here*, but it's also important to talk about devel-
oping a relationship with the *future you*, the one that's coming toward you as you read this.

This is going to seem pretty out there, but I truly believe
in this—I think about my future me all the time. Your future
you is like a small child, and each day, as you raise that child,
that future you, you have a chance to make sure the values and
beliefs you wish to have are part of this new life in the future.

How do you even start to think about a future version of
yourself when the mundane, profound problems of everyday
life seem overwhelming? Let's think about what the future
will look like in our overly technical world by looking at
what your present is.

In your present, you are bombarded by constant updates
from your friends, tasks on your to-do list, work requests and
never-ending new content from your favorite list of go-to distractions. Buried deep in this mountain of data you go through
each and every day are tiny messages from your past. Pictures,

posts, emails, text messages—they are all old versions of you. Have you ever looked for a photo and come across another photo that stopped you in your tracks and took you right back to that specific place and time? Or do you remember how magical it was the first time Facebook offered you a glimpse into your past with their On This Day feature? What about those times when you randomly come across a playlist you created months or even years ago, and just playing it sends you backward in time?

The important thing to remember about your future is that you create it by making a good past. This can be a mind bender, but a good future is usually found in how you relive your past. I'll say that again: *a good future is defined by how you relive your past.* Memories are the ground on which your future is built. Creating good memories is one of the best ways to ensure a great future—this is actually how most people look at their time.

So how do you create good memories for the future? How do you send a version of yourself to the future to be reflected upon? Well I've got good news: you already do this every day on social media and in your emails and photos.

Let's take Facebook, the easiest tool available to reprogram your future. Next time you post something on Facebook, willfully, purposefully and fully consider that one year from now, that post will show back up in your feed as a memory to review.

Go to your Facebook right now and leave yourself a note for a year from now. It can be anything really; start simple: *Dear me in the future, it's current XYZ date and it's snowing. I'm writing my first letter to you knowing that a year from today you will find this.*

Just like Doc Brown in a DeLorean speeding 88 miles per hour, a year from now your Facebook account will offer you this post to review as a memory. Take a moment to think about that. You can actually change your mood a year from now by doing this simple task right now. Yes, it's a bit of a long-term bet, but try it out. The power of talking to the future you is something that will profoundly reshape your stress levels and create some resiliency in your life.

Social media gets a bad rap. We have all seen people who live a super-glamorous life online but inside are lonely, depressed or sad. Who among us hasn't fudged the truth in an email, Instagram post or text message about the "great time" we are having. The real problem with this is how it informs our future. We forget in the future that we fudged that post, and we look back thinking, *Why can't my life be as good as it was back* then?

If you scroll through my Facebook, you'd see posts that say, "Dear Chris, it's Christmas 2024. I bet you didn't think you would make it this far! Yet here you are. Listen, today you're thinking, I'm 55 years old, and I don't know where all my time went. You're probably having doubts about your health, happiness and even your ability to get through the next 12 hours. You've done this your entire life, and you're doing it again. It seems like the first time, but I promise you it's not."

Slowly over time, you can start creating a relationship with your future self by leaving yourself notes. There are email services, text services and even old-fashioned post services that will do something similar. Yet this message-in-a-bottle part of our tech life is often overlooked. Start creating conversations with your future, now, by focusing on becoming the best ancestor you can be to yourself.

12

Self-Love:
Love Your Selfie

You're the Average of the Five Apps You Spend the Most Time With

FROM iPHONE TO wePHONE

Can our devices help us be more compassionate with ourselves, each other and even the world around us? Is the answer to coping with depression and relentless anxiety found inside our phones?

Our culture is immersed in a deep existential crisis as we close out the second decade of this century. Depression, suicide and mental illness rates are alarming across all demographics in the 2010s.

Self-love is one way to come to terms with these dark days. How do you create a compassionate relationship with your own life and story when depression, anxiety, anger or resentment sneak in? Technology actually does a really good job of helping us get used to impermanence, if we use it correctly. Mark Zuckerberg's desire for Facebook is to "make the world more open and connected." But I argue that we need to start by making ourselves more open and connected not just to each other but to ourselves.

HITTING BOTTOM

On January 3, 2015, at approximately 3:40 p.m., I was sitting inside the Regal Cinemas Green Hills 16, uncomfortably moving around in my seat as I tried to focus my attention on a movie. But my mind was racing and my heart was pounding. I stood up and whispered to my date, "I'm going to get some air, I'll be right back."

I was coming unglued. Every day since the fall of 2014, when I left Denver, I had been falling apart. I was living alone in a massive house in Tennessee, working for a big health-care company, slowly melting away physically. Everything felt new and scary.

Most days I couldn't even look in a mirror because I didn't recognize myself. My face was becoming so thin, my eyes set back in my skull. My body was changing faster than my mind.

Outside the theater, it was mystically warm for a January day, close to 61 degrees. I could feel a relentless darkness swirling around me. I'd had this feeling before, so I knew what was coming. Depression isn't a lot of what-if thinking. Depression is the loss of thought.

The darkness that accompanies my depression, which I have only felt a handful of times in my life, feels like the loss of ego, the silencing of narrative, an inescapable void, something my friend Sam refers to as "the hallow."

I found a quiet corner near the theater and phoned Natasha, my close friend and life coach. She had been by my side through breakups, job drama and ups and downs with friends for well over a decade. Natasha lives in London. I dialed her number, knowing it was late there but that she would still be awake.

"Natasha, I'm having dark thoughts." She waited for what seemed to be an hour but was only a fraction of a second.

"I understand, you have been through so much. I get them too." I didn't need to explain depression to her. I didn't need to say I wanted to kill myself or that I was lost. She could tell I was in a bad place. It started raining, sheets of water pouring from the sky, so I moved into the parking garage near the theater to continue our talk. After ten minutes, Natasha told me she loved me and we parted ways with her typical "Bye bye bye bye" tapering off to a whisper. Natasha never says good-bye, she leaves whispers of departure in your ears.

I texted apologies to my date and headed home. How was I going to make it through the night? Time had stopped and I wasn't in control of anything. In that moment, I wanted my old life back.

I got into bed and launched YouTube, but the feelings were getting worse—*what if, what if.* Then it dawned on me, *Hey, you're having what-ifs*—voices instead of a void. I quickly scrambled to launch a text file on my computer to write down what I was thinking and feeling. The part of me that understood life-logging had somehow come back online.

I'd had bad days and crazy days in the past seven years of life-logging, but I hadn't had anything like this darkness. I wanted to capture it and put it under the microscope, like a black butterfly.

GOING TO SEE BUDDHA

Realizing that my new life may have seemed perfect, by some definition or another I had created, but that my old operating system was still in control, I started doing radical things. While my body was shaping up well, I really wanted to try to get a handle on my anxiety and depression. I joined a meditation group in Nashville, started having weekly acupuncture treatments and booked a ten-day silent meditation retreat for the spring of 2015.

At my new job at Healthways, my team was moving full speed ahead on implementing a platform that would transform people's health. The media requests had slowed down but not fully stopped. And my health had never been better. I did all my work at a standing desk, I used a treadmill during the evenings in my house and I was working out with a trainer three days a week. I was finally down to my goal weight of 175 pounds.

But if I was so healthy, wealthy and wise, then why was I constantly having panic attacks alone in my mansion in the suburbs of Nashville?

The silent retreat turned out to be interesting on several levels. Spending ten straight days with 100 other people, during which no one made eye contact or spoke, ever, was a surreal experience. I mean, I knew the silent retreat would be silent. But the strangest realization, which hit me on day one, was how much we already do this in the normal world. Today, most homes, streets and places of worship are full of people not speaking to each other because they're all looking down. Luckily there were no smartphones, tablets or gaming consoles to look down at on our retreat.

I admit that taking off all my sensors was scary. My friend Taylor dropped me off after I had spent the morning "unplugging." The Fitbit that had tracked my steps and sleep for close to eight years lay on the table in front of me. My mind instantly started wondering where my steps were going to be kept.

Next, I took off my Apple Watch and powered it down. The thousands of heartbeats it had been capturing ceased to exist. My Spire sensor that normally lived under my belt capturing my respiration was placed on its charging case; the air actually left the room in some cybernetic way.

The posture belt that kept me thinking about how I sat, usually found snuggled under my waistband, lay in a bag inside my suitcase.

My mind raced. Would these things be charged when I got back? Finally, I placed my phone in airplane mode. My GPS location, social media connections, food-logging and environmental measurements all ceased to exist.

Within a few minutes, all the sensors were off my body, and the applications that controlled and kept track of my life were powered down. All the dependent logging systems started sending alerts that they couldn't connect. I'm sure the lights in my house probably blinked a few times in solidarity with my disconnected life.

I had spent years and years collecting a nonstop stream of body data, and now, it had all abruptly stopped. I had already learned very powerful lessons about listening to my body, but now it was time to listen to my head. I had to go offline.

On a silent retreat, after the "container" is created, everyone goes into silence. The first skill we learned is how to navigate without the conditioned "thank yous" and "pleases." We were told to instead replace them with a feeling of gratitude. I *felt* people's "thank you" and gave mine silently in return. As we ate our meals in silence, without looking at others, we also learned to truly notice the food we were putting into our bodies.

I started to try new things, like catching and releasing bugs instead of killing them. Turns out, your spider fears go away quickly when you watch their delight as they run away unharmed. On the retreat grounds, deer walked right up to us with no fear because we weren't a threat. Turkeys clustered in groups gazed at us calmly. In short order, we became something different, to ourselves and to others, and those around us on the retreat transformed too.

Slowly I started using nature as my sensor. Birds chirped before sunrise, and crickets sang their song before dinner. When my body became hungry, I could feel it in my blood. When I was scared, the air in my nose felt cold.

On my next-to-last day on the retreat, I had a violent panic attack while out on a walk. Somewhere on the side of a hill near George Lucas's Skywalker Ranch I started coming unglued. I had no sensors, no internet to review my symptoms. There was no one around to help me or talk to. So I did what I had been taught to do. I sat down on the ground near a rock and accepted my impending death. That's what panic feels like for me, it feels like I'm going to die. While sitting there I tried to meditate, to keep coming back to that place on Earth. Slowly, the panic lifted, though it felt like several hours. This, along with several other panic-induced meditations that year, led to a new spiritual release for me. I was at the start of a new relationship with my body and mind. One without drugs, distractions or therapy to assist me. I had to deal with myself. There was finally an "I" in my internal iPhone.

✦ ✦ ✦

In 2016, I decided it was time to start dating again, but wow, was I depressed by what I found. Although I had navigated a world of data, transformed myself and learned how to use technology to enrich my life and my feelings, the people I was meeting felt like shallow, empty versions of their technology. I joked in a Facebook post that people had turned into the hookup apps they used.

I knew there was one thing I was far from mastering: love. I had a lot to learn.

There is no app to install for finding inner peace with painful feelings. What is required is a commitment to patience with your thoughts and a devotion to self-compassion.

So I'm going to end this book with four tips that keep me grounded when mania creeps in, boost me up when depression drags me down, calm my mind when it becomes enraged and help me connect when lonely seems to be the best option.

Don't unplug, reboot.

SELF-LOVE TIPS

- ✦ **LOG AND SEARCH FOR YOUR TERROR:** Get to know you by creating a copy of your darkest moments.

- ✦ **BINGE-WATCHING HURT TO PREVENT PAIN:** Handle difficult feelings by watching other people experience them.

- ✦ **YOU ARE WHAT DRAINS YOUR PHONE BATTERY:** Learn to be resilient by tracking what apps make you happy.

- ✦ **PRACTICE IPHONE PALM READING:** Look at other people's phones to understand what we all value.

LOG AND SEARCH FOR YOUR TERROR

Get to know you by creating a copy of your darkest moments.

One of the most insidious features of anxiety and depression is their ability to make us completely reboot our mind but start it back up in a mode where it seems like everything is fixed, solid and *bad*. If there were only a way to remind yourself when these dark feelings show up that it's merely a default. The feeling of dread that accompanies anxiety is something you can't describe to anyone who has not been there. Here's how I describe panic attacks to people who have never had one: "Have you ever lost control of your car for a second on a wet road or almost been hit by someone who cut you off, and your stomach clenched and you couldn't catch your breath, your heart was pounding out of your chest and you felt like you were going to die? Now take that feeling and put it on repeat for hours and hours. That's a panic attack."

No matter if it's your first panic attack or you are on year 40 of relentless, blindsiding panic, you know that the feelings come from nowhere and they are always brand new. The feelings lie to you and tell you that this time is different, that this time they won't go away, that you're going to go crazy, die or lose everything.

Technology's main utility during these times of sheer terror usually is that you can endlessly search for the symptoms of heart attacks and strokes or information on depression, anxiety or even suicide.

Unfortunately, when you use technology to look up symptoms, if you're like me, you become the symptoms. When you're a digital hypochondriac, using technology when you are suffering is anything but helpful. Then if you somehow make it out of the rabbit hole of WebMD's checklist of the physical symptoms, it is hard not to be hyper-vigilant about checking your physical monitors. How is your heart rate? You have an entire body to search and read about. Digital health isn't for the faint of heart. One of the things that sometimes helps is to distract yourself.

If only there were a way to search within your own history and experience? A way to look back at previous episodes of anxiety, depression and fear?

Once in the middle of a panic attack I came across an old journal entry I had written while in the midst of a world-class panic attack. Reading it, I remembered writing it, and slowly my panic decreased. Within a few minutes I felt better.

What if we could find information on the web about our past as easily as we could about celebrities, science and history? I decided to record all my episodes of depression, panic and rage. The physical symptoms, the feelings, the thoughts. I called this my "Wikipedia of Fear." The process is pretty simple. You break the magical hold that panic has on you when you reread your own words describing your own past experience.

It's best to create your fear Wikipedia when you're not in the middle of an attack. Simply recall a time when you had a panic attack or depressive episode and start listing your symptoms. Break them down into physical symptoms, mental symptoms, thoughts and behaviors. Keep them in NotePad on your phone or even as something printed in your wallet. Next time you start to feel any of these dark feelings, grab your phone and pull up the note. Review the symptoms and compare them to how you are feeling. Seriously, this really helps. Your checklist in your Wikipedia of Fear is the first sign to yourself that you're going to be ok. You've been here before and you lived!

As you become more adept with this coping skill, you can add to your symptom checklists in the middle of an attack. The good news is that doing this helps create a really good distraction for yourself. You become an observer of your own episode.

Below is an attack I had in 2015, as dictated into my phone.

JANUARY 5, 2015
5 P.M. TO 11 P.M.

Physical:

- *Cold hands*
- *Cold Feet*
- *Shaking*
- *Get warm under the covers*
- *Stomach gets sick*
- *Can't sit still*
- *Dry mouth*

- *Legs shaky but can't sit still, I felt this way in the hospital when they were monitoring me*

Behaviors:

- *Keep getting up and walking around*
- *Can't stop looking up things on my phone*
- *Go to drink water then spit it out*

Mental:

- *Racing thoughts*
- *Can't focus*
- *Worried about the future*
- *Can't keep a sentence together*
- *Can't focus*
- *Thoughts of doom*
- *Thoughts of shame*

Thoughts:

- *I'm thinking about my boyfriend*
- *I'm worried I'll look foolish in front of friends*
- *I'm worried I will lose everything*
- *I'm worried about the project at work*
- *I'm worried about my ex*
- *I have been reading internet horror stories*
- *I am ashamed of my behavior on New Year's Eve*
- *I am close to three months off lower Klonopin with no issues until after New Year's Eve*
- *I'm worried I'll be back in my 20s and get so anxious and sad that I end up in a hospital*

As you can see, this anxiety attack was terrifying for me, but somehow becoming the historian of my attack served as an important way for me to look at these events more objectively. Now each time I have an attack, I have a clear map of what is happening and what I can expect.

Sometimes even with the best list of symptoms, your mind will still tell you, "Hey, this is a neat trick, but dude, you're going to die this time." Our minds are such assholes sometimes.

To that end, I've made it a point to list every panic or depression I have had, and I keep this list handy. The timeline of my life's major anxiety and depressive moments serves as a reminder that I've come through this before.

Below is part of my "List of Places" that I use when I need to be brought back to the present moment.

- Remember going to the hospital when you were 16 in the middle of the night? May 1985
- Remember crossing the bridge on the way to New Jersey? 1989
- Remember leaving Central Station? February 1991
- Remember Rob Ward's mother giving me a book after an attack? 1992
- Remember going to the freezer at Highs? March 1993
- Remember going to Julie's having a panic attack? 1996

It goes all the way up to the present day. These lists or journals you keep on your phone, laptop or table are a great way to start to manage your anxiety, panic, depression or other difficult feelings. Don't limit yourself to just anxiety and depression. Keep lists for anger, loneliness, rage, envy and greed. Really, there is no feeling you can't map, document and relive.

BINGE-WATCHING HURT TO PREVENT PAIN

Handle difficult feelings by watching other people experience them.

Some of my most provocative cybernetic mind hacks were things I found by accident without data but kept secret until now or only shared in a workshop. This next tip is one of those hacks. During a particularly vicious depressive episode, I was Google-searching suicide. (Yeah, like I said earlier, sometimes technology is not helpful.) I stumbled on someone who posted a video about depression, and just like every other time, I got lost in the maze of YouTube. I looked at the suggested videos and one caught my eye—the title was something along the lines of "I want to die, I'm so depressed." Reluctantly, I clicked on the video and started watching this person, someone who was devoid of emotion, talk about their symptoms and how they probably were going to kill themselves.

My depression lifted and my mood lightened. I wasn't alone in the world. There were other people like me. For a moment though, I was caught off guard. How could watching someone fall apart cancel out my own despondent feelings? What was going on?

A week later, I had a panic episode, so I tried it again. I searched for and watched videos of people having anxiety attacks, and within a few moments, sure enough, the panic videos canceled out my own anxiety.

Finding a way to feel less alone when those episodes hit me was world-changing. I doubled down on my newfound digital Prozac, creating playlists on YouTube of all the different emotions I tended to get weighed down by: depression, panic, rage and so on. To this day, I still use these videos when my own symptom lists aren't doing the trick.

These playlists on my "Netflix of Darkness" have also created a new routine that helped me overcome one of my darkest emotions, the one that always leads to panic and depression: anger. Anger to me is the gateway drug to shame, and shame always takes me straight to depression and anxiety. I needed a way to inoculate myself against anger, so I started watching public freak-out videos on a popular internet community site called Reddit. These videos helped me see how ridiculous anger is and helped me spot it in myself.

The best way to avoid or lessen those unwanted feelings that plague us is to be more mindful of our behaviors, particularly the bad ones, and create more meaningful relationships ourselves. Our devices don't have to be our hiding place, where we avoid other people or even ourselves; instead, we can use them as bridges to create deep meaningful relationships both with ourselves and with the people around us.

YOU ARE WHAT DRAINS YOUR PHONE BATTERY
Learn to be resilient by tracking what apps make you happy.

The mindful cyborg knows that his understanding of happiness can be found in the battery consumption section of his or her phone. Within every smartphone is a section, usually in settings, that will show you which apps are using the most battery. It will be sorted by last 24 hours or last seven days. This list is a powerful map for your emotions. For instance, if you have been feeling better than normal, chances are the apps that are listed in the last 24 hours are radically different from the apps you used in the past seven days.

The opposite is also true: if you're feeling blue, your app usage has probably changed. Next time you're feeling great, take a screenshot of your battery percentages and keep track of your happy apps—whatever you've been spending more time with lately has obviously kept you feeling great.

More importantly, if you start feeling a bit low, pull up that list of happy apps and start forcing yourself to use the apps that bring you joy. For me, I'm most happy when using Evernote, Maps and Calendar, and I'm most depressed and sad when on Twitter, Fitbit and Facebook. When times get tough, I avoid my sad apps and focus on my happy apps. The answers are right in front of you, and your tech can help you find them.

PRACTICE IPHONE PALM READING
Look at other people's phones to understand what we all value.

In a world where we are told we are not good humans because we can't stop looking down at our phones, I want to end the section on self-care with how to connect to others while keeping our technology close at hand.

For close to five years, I have been doing iPhone palmistry for strangers at bars and conferences around the world. Seriously, conferences pay me thousands of dollars to sit inside a fortune-teller booth I keep and ship to events. iPhone palmistry? #WTF is that?

It's exactly what the name implies: I do a psychic reading via your iPhone and answer questions about your life and future. But how do I do it, and why am I encouraging you to try it out with your friends?

First why. It's simple: there is no faster route to getting to know someone—a friend, family member or peer—than by handling their phone. Our phones are the most intimate tool we have, our entire lives are stored in them. So how does iPhone palmistry work?

You need to be respectful. (In this age of consent, it is wise to make sure the person is comfortable with what you're doing!) For example, you shouldn't open any apps, you should only look at the case and the home screen. You don't want to exploit someone's most vulnerable moments in a reading. By setting this guideline, you create some trust between you and the person you're reading.

Your job is just to examine the phone and learn what you can about the person. I often start by just looking at what type of phone it is, or if it has a case. Something simple. Talk about what you are feeling as you look at the phone.

Remember, the goal of this experience is to create deep and meaningful conversations. Don't dig too deeply; the goal is to provoke your partner into wanting to share more about their life with you.

If you find a friend willing to test this game out, after sharing the guidelines, trade phones and take a few minutes to examine their phone, case and home screen. Then the person being read sits quietly, without interrupting, while the reader reviews what they found in their partner's phone. This is where the magic happens.

Here are some things I look for on phones and how I interpret them:

Physical Device:

- iPhone or Android. Android users tend to be very tech-centered people, hardcore geeks, the coders of the world, whereas iPhone users generally seem to be more focused on aesthetic quality and, sometimes, status.
- Telltale signs of age and wear. Does your palmistry partner have the latest and greatest phone, or is it beat-up, with a cracked screen and dented edges? Phones with a lot of wear and tear, scrapes and cracked screens speak to people who are sporty, outdoor types. (You'll find a lot more busted smartphones in the pockets of the average REI consumer than someone shopping at the local party store. Strange how that works!)
- The case or screen protector, or lack thereof. Is the case almost impervious to damage, with a screen protector? Is the device inside a giant bag? If so, you can almost always

expect someone who has been burned a few times or was raised in an environment where security might not have been the first order of the day. How we protect our devices speaks to how we watch after our hearts. Strangely enough, if you spend any time in Scandinavia, you will see most people do not protect their phones at all: no cases, covers or screen protectors. (Perhaps the sense of safety they feel living in a socialist state extends to their technology?)

Inside the Machine:

- Lock-screen wallpapers are always where we present the face we wish to be known for to the world. Family members, pets, vacation photos and art adorn our lock screens. The magic to the lock-screen photo isn't found on the lock screen, but on the home screen. People who take time to have different lock-screen photos from home-screen photos tend to be more complex individuals; they separate work and life and do a good job balancing.

- Home screens are where we find the soul of our friends and mates. Home screens can be full of icons, nested folders, organized by activity type or even app icon color. Each home screen is a glimpse into the mind of the person you're reading. My favorite people to read don't have a lot of icons on their home screen. I've found that when you don't fill up your home screen with things to do, you're generally a more peaceful person. The exact opposite of our Zen friends would be people who fill their home screens with folders full of apps, without a single place to add anything. These people will probably never let you read their phones, as they are too busy planning their next icon rearrangement. The real cyborg deviants among us are the people who willfully and purposefully leave their home screen alone with the default icons straight from the factory neatly lined up.

The cyborg equivalent of the white picket fence. Often these people hide behind "I don't care about my phone," and they stuff all their sins on their second or third screen.

- Notification badges or onscreen alerts. You'll always meet that one person with 3,000 unread email messages and 500 text messages awaiting a reply. There is something comforting to these people about needing to be needed and being reminded of this often.

In this game, let your intuition guide you. Then share your findings in a safe, open and honest way. You'll find that some people are unable to stay silent while you read their phone. They will want to correct you with each observation. Patiently explain that the goal of the exercise is to explore the insights you've found on the phone and you can't be influenced with additional information. Once the reading is done, allow your partner to respond. Then switch and prepare to be read!

Our phones give us a chance to explain our values, rituals and love, without the nasty overhead of an awkward fishing conversation or the downright insidious social media stalking. I've found that families, husbands and wives, coworkers—so many people—have no idea who they are really sitting next to every day. Often, these exercises create a new level of trust and empathy.

THE FUTURE

We need to start being more open about our technology use and consumption. Explore what it means to you and what it means to the important people in your life. Trust me, if your browser history is important to Google, your Facebook friends are important to Facebook and your location is important to Apple, your life could and should be that important to you and your friends.

You don't need to understand the latest technology or services to talk about how you use them or why. The conversations we lost to technology can be rekindled by talking about how we use the technology.

There are apps to help you do everything; taking the time to look at a normal app in a new way will help you learn about who you are. I never intended to use alarms for mindfulness, maps for love, notes for journals or videos for group therapy. Get to know who you are by examining the reflection coming back at you in the apps you use. It's like fixing your digital hair, but with much more profound implications for your well-being.

Big Lover:
I Love You, Don't Block Me

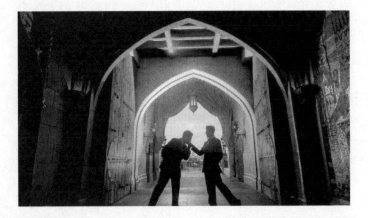

*"Stop valuing your schedule and start scheduling
your values."*

—Chris Dancy

As my technology stack grew and morphed, I struggled to find love.

Today it's increasingly hard to feel like you belong or fit into anyone's schedule. The feelings of isolation and loneliness that technology can leave us with often overwhelm us into believing that maybe the good old days of going on an actual date with someone you couldn't Google-stalk before meeting them are long gone.

Sherry Turkle of MIT has been proselytizing her own brand of digital dualism since the early 2010s. In her bestselling book *Alone Together*, she begs us to engage in genuine and authentic conversations. As a gay man nearing the age of 50, it was obvious to me I was falling into the same trap of wistful nostalgia, yearning for dates that didn't involve apps.

If you pull back the veil from all the sensational headlines, you find love and intimacy are thriving in the tweets, snaps and hashtags of today's cyborgs.

I use the word *cyborg* on purpose, because I think it's important to think about what life is like with cyborgs. What is a cyborg? According to Wikipedia, "the term cyborg is not the same thing as bionic, bio-robot or android. Cyborg is an organism that has restored function or enhanced abilities due to the integration of some artificial component or technology that relies on some sort of feedback."

Who on Earth doesn't have restored function or enhanced abilities due to integration with technology? This is every single person carrying a smartphone. You can now translate any language to any other. You can look up plants to avoid eating something poisonous. Our phones in some ways have made us superhuman. As far as feedback, who on Earth isn't hopelessly reprogrammed by the feedback loops of our social media?

So we're different. But that's ok, isn't it? Let's try to slow down the dangerous language lamenting the fact that we are not human any more. We are cyborgs, and that means learning to love and think a bit differently.

The title of this book is *Don't Unplug*, and if you truly feel there is value in staying connected to find digital salvation, you will want to learn how to love and be loved in this age of hyper-connection.

In 1996, when I first met my longtime partner, Doug, on an AOL Instant Messenger chat, I never imagined a world where people didn't or couldn't find love without the internet. But two decades later, that's exactly where we are. For me, by the beginning of 2016, my fear that my body, life and health were evolving so fast that I could not keep up were starting to abate.

The disdain I felt for people who were not working in flow had started to subside. We all know that type-A person who talks of body hacking or becomes obsessed with health and fitness. (I was probably pretty intolerable.) But at long last, my battle to attain perfection, or perhaps me giving up that battle, had finally led me to a more peaceful place, or at least to moments of continuous satisfaction.

Was it going to be possible to find another mindful cyborg in this new world? Digital relationships were not new for me, but life had evolved a lot since online dating took off. Dating now is about surveillance, algorithms and big money.

Algorithmically arranged marriages are becoming the norm. How else do you explain Tinder or Grindr? The apps learn what we like in a person, then present those users to us. Anyone who is on a dating app will tell you it's about your profile picture or your bio, or probably both. It's about being authentic but not needy, being sexy but not fake—no obvious filter use. You should be career-motivated but not obsessed. Don't post your credit score or bank balance (yes, people do that).

For months in the beginning of 2016, I tried to find some-one, but I was having no luck. I knew what I wanted. There had to be an immediate attraction, but not so much that I was ob-sessively jealous. Age was obviously a factor I was not going to be able to get around. Additionally, dating outside of my gen-eration wasn't going to work. If I went up a generation, I might need to put my partner in hospice care on our tenth anniver-sary; if I went down a generation, I would have someone else's student debt to pay off.

None of the dating sites were giving me the data I wanted. But I soon found that if I paid up for the premium version of the services, going from $10 to $100 per month, I could get access to the raw feed of humanity. Perhaps it won't come as a surprise that I was concerned about getting access to the raw data behind the curtain.

I could filter out anyone who was not into safe sex, who was below 5′4″ or over 220 pounds. I could review my super likes and even push myself to the top of someone else's stack of candidates. With each new criteria, the number of eligible dates grew smaller and smaller.

I had some successful dates in early 2016—I even met some-one I fell in heavy with, but there was always a catch. Age was the number-one thing, but sometimes my own bleeding heart would get in the way. I'd find someone to save or fix. I jokingly used to say, "I have to save guys from the future or restore their past." But no one was ticking all my boxes. I wanted a clean-cut geek, age 25 to 43, height 5′8″ to 6′4″, weight 150 to 210 pounds, with a few other vital likes and dislikes checked off on my list. How hard would it be to find this guy?

Then, on May 31, 2016, I checked my phone, and there in the middle of my screen was a single photo. My heart started racing. He had apparently made it past every single one of my filters. Could there actually be a perfect person for me right here in Nashville? But with Bill Gates as my witness, all my filters had found a perfect match within 20 miles of me.

✦ ✦ ✦

Mid-20s, schoolteacher, into family, single, looking to date, handsome, like a Latin Clark Kent. My heart was pounding. I sent him a screenshot of my filter and a note about how he had hit every category. I think I used the word "perfection."

Luckily that didn't scare him away. He messaged me back and for 48 hours we communicated nonstop. His name was Fernando and he was visiting with his family from Houston, Texas. He was a high school drama teacher and definitely a momma's boy. His messages were written with caution but his GIFs and emojis were sent with reckless abandon. It was as if I knew him already; he spoke a kind of cyborg language all itself.

(It would be some time before it dawned on me that far too many millennials have emotional cores based around internet memes and YouTube reaction videos.)

We kept trying but failing to meet in person. On the last day before he was to leave, I took matters into my own hands. I knew from his messages that he was staying in Lewisburg, Tennessee. Lewisburg is a town of 11,000 people and one Walmart. How hard was it going to be for me to find one guy from Texas?

I jumped in my truck and sped off. The automatic sensor was beeping and chirping wildly as I hard braked and suddenly accelerated like a crazy person. The 35-minute drive to Lewisburg was nerve-wracking. I arrived just as the sun was about to set, raced into the Walmart and bought some flowers.

I looked at my phone and took a deep breath. Here goes.

"Hey, me here, guess where I am?" I texted, then watched as the three dots came up on my screen as Fernando started texting me back. I flipped over to the info portion of the text message and selected "Share Location," then selected "Share Indefinitely." A map appeared on my screen, then Fernando stopped texting. Oh God. Was he freaking out that some crazy guy had tracked him down and was looking for him? I waited for what felt like an eternity. No texts. I had blown it.

I heard a sound behind me. I turned around to see a car pulling up to the empty Goodwill parking lot I was standing in. The sun was starting to set and the lights of the parking lot had just come on. My eyes focused. The car was from Texas. Fernando had used the location to drive to me.

He parked next to my truck and walked toward me, confident, eyes of chocolate, a smile like sunlight. I held the bouquet of flowers out to him. He smiled broadly and without a word, we hugged. I started to tear up. (Why was I crying? I didn't even know this guy.) Then the explosions started. Literal explosions. It was the night of July 3 and the locals were testing their Fourth of July goodies. I looked at Fernando and started smiling. He could see the tears in my eyes; we both acknowledged the fireworks without a word and then kissed. More fireworks. As I pulled out onto the back roads of Tennessee, I sent him a photo of the sunset with one single line: "This is for you."

Fernando and I long-distance-dated for months, often spending hours on the phone or jumping on planes to go see each other. Within six months we were living together. Everything I had worked for was aligning, my 0 had found a 1.

✦ ✦ ✦

What I learned about Fernando in the first year of our relationship was everything I needed to know about technology and love. I learned to send love through my devices. I learned when to use technology to show love and when to leave it alone.

In the spring of 2017, I was teaching my "Love and Technology" workshop to a group of professionals at GroupM in Stockholm, Sweden. The people in the room ranged in age from early twenties to mid-fifties. They all sat nervously in a circle as I talked openly about my relationship with Fernando, my friends, family and feelings.

Slowly through the three-hour session, they opened up about their partners, spouses and lovers. Everyone felt lonely and they were blaming technology.

Originally, I wanted to write a book just about spirituality and love, but no one wanted that, they wanted the whole "Chris Dancy" story. When I signed the contract to turn my decade-long experiment into a book, I wasn't in love—in fact, I was in the absence of love, I was in self-neglect, but damn I had some good numbers to show for it, on the scale, in the bank and in hours logged at work.

I can only now share with you these tips on how to love, in spite of technology, because like the rest of my lessons, this one came just in time.

Don't unplug, love more.

BIG LOVER TIPS

✦ **EMOTIONS 2.0:** The technology of feelings.

✦ **ORWELLIAN SURVEILLANCE:** Opt into surveillance for the sake of love.

✦ **CYBORG LUNCH-BOX NOTES:** Leave love notes in the cloud.

✦ **DIGITAL SKIN-WALKING:** How switching phones will create a new level of patience and empathy for the busy lovers in our life.

✦ **LOVE GPS:** Love in the future.

EMOTIONS 2.0

The technology of feelings.

It was probably sometime in 2014 that I noticed that it had become more common to post an animated GIF in reaction to a tweet than to spend an entire 11 seconds composing an exhausting 140-character response. The 2000s were exhausting me. When I learned that "xo" had been replaced by the outrageously da Vinci–esque "<3," I nearly cried. Who was deciding that the keyboard versions of my emotions needed upgrading?

In the 2010s, our digital emotions evolved at warp speed. Our vocabulary of text-based emotions or emoticons had morphed into the Tumblr-animated GIFs of the 2000s and quickly filled our social streams with emojis, hashtags and biometrics. In less than ten years, from 2008 to 2018, we went from people sending ":)" to fully animated characters of ourselves (Apple calls them animoji), perfectly 3D face-mapped and sent with voice to our loved ones.

But instead of throwing up our hands and opting out of communication entirely, perhaps there are ways we can use this way of expressing emotions to help our relationships. We need to be perfectly honest with ourselves about what constitutes real love and togetherness. While I would much prefer to be holding someone's hand, it is not any more real than when you are across the world from a loved one, falling asleep while looking at each other over Skype or FaceTime.

Love transcends technology. Let's stop the shame and the fear that we are not truly loving each other. We are doing the best we can, and that is how love should be defined.

First rule of texting: never text what you can save for later. Seriously, text doesn't have to be your running brain dump, and it certainly should never be used for big talks. Text itself holds the promise of short messages of love and support. I have stopped using text messages for time-sensitive requests. This goes against conventional wisdom, but I wanted to remove the anxiety of waiting for a text back.

Text messaging, for me anyway, became a way to say, "I love you, I'm proud of you, I'm thinking of you." I'll share my location when I arrive someplace safely. I'll send a photo from the day, a screenshot of something I saw. Text messages are the refrigerator door of my heart, and what I put up there for my loved ones are the things that inspire hope.

The future of text messages holds even more intimate types of messaging now that we wear our technology. Today we can use text-based gestures, draw pictures and smiley faces and even use our finger to spell out "love." Today you can actually tell your Apple iPhone to send a message with "gentle effect" and it will play the text on my partner's screen with a subtle motion, almost like the text is breathing. Or I can use a "slam effect" to remind my partner of my confidence in their big day.

Although text effects in our messages may not work on all phones, GIFs and emojis do. There are entire keyboard replacements for these new emotional expressions. Celebrating a big trip? Send a Wizard of Oz GIF of Dorothy heading down the Yellow Brick Road. GIFs do what words can't—they paint a thousand emotions.

If we were really honest about our emergent cyborgnetic emotions, we could see that kids today use memes as their shared cultural responses to pop culture. Think about that: we have evolved into mini Andy Warhols, appropriating Boomer, Gen X and Gen Y culture into temporal touchstones to express the sentiments of an entire population.

This, my friends, is a provocative time to be human, as we embrace tools that express new sets of emotion. And these tools are just getting started. Facebook has now launched text-based flourishes where you type "congrats" or "xoxo" and the screen becomes a "link" to a set of screen explosions of confetti or hearts. So next time a friend or loved one sends you an emoji or a GIF, remember that these aren't just a passing fad of a keyboard-addicted generation, these are the emergent emotions for a new way of love. You're being kissed for the first time. (I kissed a cyborg and I liked it.)

ORWELLIAN SURVEILLANCE
Opt into surveillance for the sake of love.

Digital love in today's world is, let's be honest, purposeful, willful, over-the-top surveillance. Most relationships have always had a certain amount of Orwellian surveillance built into them, but with today's tools, it can be taken to a whole new level. Normally people would assume this means that you "stalk" or "creep" on your partner's online activity, but that's not what I'm proposing. Surveillance can be used for good. What I want you to do is to create a relationship with your partner where technology acts as a mediator between both of you and your busy lives.

How does this work? Well, it can be as simple as saving screenshots as moments of love. With today's phones, screenshots are a high art. Tools are built-in to annotate, edit and update photos. These digital scrapbook entries are a beautiful way to show your partner how much you care. You can even place all these screenshots in a shared photo album; then, as new screenshots are placed in the folder, you both would receive alerts letting you know that the other person had added a new image, comment or update to the photos.

This very simple process can create a revolutionary dialogue for both of you about what you value, as individuals and as a couple. More importantly, it serves as a reminder to both of you of what you share and what you believe in for your future together.

Instagram, Facebook and Twitter are all common communication tools for millions of couples around the planet. They are, sadly, the source of so much shame and blame, but they also are a source of hope and delight, a treasure trove of material for strangers and lovers alike to plunder like the cyborg pirates of the new world. Yet if you know where to look, there is the possibility of something deeper and much more spiritual within these tools.

Often our social media represents a snapshot of what we love, value and treasure in a moment. Like all feelings, these moments are transitory, an ephemeral projection of the hour or day we are having. Yet, after a few weeks, these treasured memories become the worthless castoffs of an algorithm that no longer finds value in these items. Are our memories still golden after the likes and hearts stop coming in?

By taking time each week to review your partner's old posts, you can in essence send digital kisses. Within the blink of an eye, your partner will get an update that a post was liked. When your lover logs in, they will be instantly transported to a time in recent memory that the machines in our lives have forgotten about, but that you, with your love, have not.

This digital love hack is powerful, and I encourage you to try it. The best ones are when your partner is having a problem in life and they need indirect guidance. When they are struggling with work or health, liking old photos where work and health were in flux and they successfully navigated that difficult time is a great way to offer support. A "renewed like" instills confidence. Your online history is full of love, compassion and grace. Find your heart even in the darkest of hours by looking beyond the algorithms life offers us and becoming the historian of your own kindness.

CYBORG LUNCH-BOX NOTES
Leave love notes in the cloud.

Remember back when your mom would leave you a note in your lunch? Or what about when you would go to the medicine cabinet and find a sticky note from your partner that just said, "I love you"? We live in a time where creating these forget-me-nots is easier than ever. Some of the most beautiful moments in a day come when we get a text message from our lover with words of encouragement.

Let's take apart our smartphone and repurpose it as a digital lunch box, one that we are going to fill with notes of encouragement and love for our partners and loved ones. Text messages work best for this type of thing, and often we forget to use this vital heart-healing tool for just that. Often, I will schedule a reminder for myself on a big day for someone I love, and about 10 minutes before that big meeting, sad goodbye or long trip, I get a note reminding me to reach out to my friend with words of encouragement.

This is the exact opposite of the garish social media outcry of birthday well wishes. It doesn't have the resentment of the forced reminder systems that give away the private data of our lives, and it's not the mock anniversaries of our relationships with our friends or the milestones that are algorithmically conjured up in our feeds. No, these reminders that you create and send are the truly private feeds of our most admired, loved partners.

Next time your friend or loved one has a tough event coming up, take time to send support before and after. Yet there are so many ways we can go beyond just a time for support.

What about a place for support? There's an app for that too. Today's artificial intelligences, Siri, Ok Google and Cortana, all have location awareness. I can create a simple location-based reminder: "Hey Siri, remind me when I get home that Fernando loves me." Now after a long day of work, when I pull up in the driveway, my watch vibrates and the message "Fernando loves you" pops up on my wrist. Wow, the power of *here* is so much more compelling than the power of *now*.

This simple relationship hack is a lunch-box note to myself, from myself, to focus on love, on what's truly important to me. If you're an extreme life hacker, a term I've never liked, tools like Foursquare allow you to check into places together. Now when your partner goes to the grocery store or the hair salon, you can leave notes of encouragement or love.

Finally, it's not a new phenomenon to have a lock-screen or wallpaper photo of your partner, but what you can do with these images is new. A real cyborg Romeo knows that within each new upgrade to our technology is the opportunity to upgrade our love. Long gone are the days where our photos are static, staged moments of intimacy. Today's photos are alive with motion. Apple calls these "live photos" and Google calls them "motion photos." Now when you take a photo, the camera can save a half-second before and after the picture. To access the hidden movement in today's photos, you simply press and hold your screen to reveal the secret dance of staged smiles. In this small piece of time, unfrozen technology is the promise of the coolest lunch-box notes you can create.

Next time you take a selfie, snap the photo, but right after the shutter release quickly blow a kiss at the screen. The result: a really nice selfie that reveals a secret kiss when your partner presses the screen.

DIGITAL SKIN-WALKING

> How switching phones will create a new level of patience and
> empathy for the busy lovers in our life.

It's hard to be in love today. We are busy, schedules are tight and distraction is a mistress with seductive powers beyond anything we can find on Pornhub. Is it possible to be tethered both to our devices and to our partners? Can we balance our online and offline time?

We live in a culture where half the world is demanding that we put our devices down, be present, be in the moment. We all know that sick feeling we get when we sneak to the bathroom to check for an email from work. Or the sinking feeling we get when our spouse notices us touching our device for the thirtieth time this hour. So how do we lower the shame threshold of using technology while simultaneously creating a deeper, more thoughtful relationship with our partners?

Simple: digital skin-walking. In certain Native American cultures, it was believed that you could morph into another creature by wearing its pelt. You become the wolf by wearing the wolf's hide; you could forge a deeper sympathy for nature and the creatures around you from living in this hyper-empathetic state.

In essence, for a short time each day, just to practice empathy, I encourage you to switch devices with your partner. There, I said it, and I'll say it again. I want you and your partner to actually switch phones. When the phone rings, a text message comes in or an email is received, you, acting as your partner, review the message and then share it with your spouse. "Hey, your mom just texted and wanted to know when we will arrive next week." Or maybe I get an email from a company about a consulting engagement I'm involved in. "Chris, you just got an email from Microsoft, they want to know if you can change your talk from one hour to 45 minutes." Then you discuss it and respond for your partner.

This type of behavior is, oddly enough, groundbreaking for couples. At first it will really throw you off, because it seems strange and unnatural, but soon the magic of "becoming" your partner's phone starts to reveal itself. Frustration with your lover's relationship with devices becomes an awareness of the dependencies in their life beyond you. You probably hear about that annoying coworker of theirs over dinner, but it's a lot different when you have to reply to their emails. You could imagine being friends with your partner's yoga teacher, but it's a lot different to see her posts on Facebook every hour inviting you to the next aromatherapy meetup.

Taking time to become your partner on their device, you start to develop a level of appreciation for the deep commitments they have to the world outside of your home. Traditionally, partners share finances, legal responsibilities and sometimes schedules, but it stops there. Why would we choose to only share the nightmare of bills and the burden of legalities and leave the rest of our lives concealed from each other? This type of radical acceptance of our partners hits at the roots of distraction in the world today.

Just once, put on the digital skin of the wild animal you call your partner and become them, inhabit their world. Then, the next time they are hopelessly lost in their phone screen, you'll have a level of empathy that will heal the wounded pride of screaming for a swipe right.

LOVE GPS
Love in the future.

No one downloads an app, they download a habit. This concept of downloading a habit is one of the most disruptive things that is happening to everyone I know.

For what it's worth, technology didn't upgrade me, the habits technology created in me upgraded me. Data didn't solve my behavior issues, it revealed them. Devices didn't make my intimacy distracted, it deepened how I look for love. As the world rockets toward my vision for love, I thought it would be good to review how I love today.

One of the first big purchases Fernando and I made together was a Tesla Model X. This semiautonomous solid-state vehicle is symbolic of the world we all will occupy. Electric cars, unlike their fossil-fuel siblings, need recharging, just like our bodies. Your Tesla needs a full eight-hour charge in the garage each night, a lot like our bodies require seven to eight hours of sleep. It also means that on a road trip, you need to stop for at least one hour to recharge.

So your car becomes a type of lifestyle and a new set of habits. For some new owners of a Tesla, the car creates a condition called "range anxiety." Range anxiety is the fear that your car will run out of battery and you won't be near a charger. We all have experienced this type of anxiety when our phones or laptops get low and there's no outlet nearby.

Deciding to take a road trip means forced planning, forced downtime, forced thought. Now when Fernando and I go on a trip, we know that every three to four hours we will have to stop for at least one hour to recharge the car. Gone are the days where we raced from place to place, got off at an exit to jam a burger in our mouths and got back on the road. Now we have to stop, and it has become our chance to explore, connect and see the world we used to zoom right past.

Tesla is the most mindful piece of technology ever created and gives me a great deal of hope. Yet we are just beginning to look at the deeper connections with autonomous cars and love. One of the most exciting features in these cars of tomorrow is that they will completely auto-steer, change lanes and slow down when we are on trips.

The very first time Fernando and I were in the car alone and having it drive for us, we used the moment to celebrate by doing something you don't get to experience in cars traveling at 70 miles per hour. We kissed. I took my hands off the wheel, looked at Fernando and said, "I love you." Then I leaned over and kissed him.

In that moment, the future of love and technology was revealed to me. There we were, speeding down Route 65 just south of Nashville, Selena Gomez blaring, and we were kissing. Isn't this what we should focus on the next time someone says that driverless cars will kill people? Couldn't we also say, "Yeah, but we will kiss more"?

✦ ✦ ✦

We don't need a virtual reality, we have a reality. We don't need innovation, we need compassion. We don't need to fix the problems of the world with technology, we need to fix technology with our human spirit.

I hope I live long enough to see a world where we all kiss more in autonomous cars, where we download memories and relive the good times and bad. I want to share my love in any way that connects it to someone I care about. While I don't know if I will ever see this time, I know my data will, because I didn't unplug; I kept going and so should you.

Acknowledgments

My life wouldn't be possible without the love and support from my parents, **Charles and Priscilla Dancy**. While they both have moved on from this world, the good, bad and awkward they instilled within me moves me through my life. My family was a reality show in real life.

Like most teenagers, my life was shaped by music, and I can say without a doubt my relationship with **Michael Jackson** has been a strong influence in my life. Michael understood media, attention and the dance of human novelty. Michael Jackson was an internet trend in human form.

My formative years as an adult were guided by several business leaders who forever evolved my definition of "work" and helped me understand my value and potential. First was **Helena HoTseung**, who upon selling her business gave every employee part of the proceeds, showing me how leadership is created and maintained to the end. Next, **Ashley Leonard**, who grew a small team of engineers into a global business, always remembered his employees were the product and reminded me to "keep going." Billionaire cloud pioneer **Fred Luddy**, who, when the entire HR team said "he's not worth it," stayed the course and believed in me. **Kia Behnia**, who had the vision to see that my understanding of mobile computing could disrupt an entire industry and relentlessly challenged me to keep moving forward. And finally, **Ben Leedle**: Ben had a vision for populations and health before many people understood either. Ben created more careers and launched more successful businesses than anyone I know. Ben Leedle is a hero and should be regarded as one. These business leaders were the platforms to my success, and without them, I would not have achieved so much.

My health is a large part of this book, and therefore it would be incredulous not to mention the providers who shaped me physically and mentally. First, **Dr. William Alford**, who got me through several drug rehabs, bouts of depression and a physical body that was nearing death. Second, **Dr. Robert Beck**, who defined modern digital health by always stopping to talk to me about my health and remind me that I was "not my numbers." While healthcare and wellness should be human rights, your body is a temple.

Like so many medical providers through the years who nursed my body back to health, two therapists helped me work with my thoughts and mind. First was **Dr. Sally Winston**, who treated me for anxiety disorder when I was hospitalized in my early 20s. Dr. Winston regularly helped me address my thoughts and reminded me how to work with my mind. Finally, **Dr. Ellen Lewis**, who helped ween me off of 20 years of antidepressants and benzodiazepines. As my body and life improved, Dr. Lewis was singularly charged with helping me learn "Skills over Pills." Make therapy, medication and your mind an ally, for only your perception can shape your reality.

My spiritual journey has been shaped by so many people, from my first visit to church to my last Buddhist retreat at

Spirit Rock. I'd like to take a moment to thank the teachers who have genuinely shaped my mind and whose wisdom forever graces the Earth: **Jon Kabat-Zinn** and **Pema Chodron**. To that end, my enduring gratitude to the global Shambhala Buddhist community for always having a place for me to sit and do nothing. If you don't have 10 minutes to meditate, you need to meditate for 20 minutes.

A book with this much technology should have an extensive technology acknowledgment section, but for me, I don't feel the need. As a young professional, I worshipped **Bill Gates** and dreamed of working at Microsoft. Bill Gates has proven by creating technology that he can reshape the world to be healthier and kinder with the Bill and Melinda Gates Foundation. Finally, **Tim Berners-Lee**, who gave us this new world we call the internet and to this day fights tirelessly for all of our freedoms: May you all never unplug.

Last, I'm often asked, "Who do you read, study, etc.?" I never am quite sure how to answer this question as I go out of my way not to be biased or influenced by any particular school of thought until I have formed my opinion. To that end though there are a few historical figures who I have taken time to study, read and re-read: **Douglas Rushkoff, Alan Watts, Terence McKenna, Søren Kierkegaard, Andy Warhol, Antoni Gaudí, Carl Jung, Robert Anton Wilson, Alvin Toffler, Winston Churchill and Viktor E. Frankl.**

Finally, thank you to my husband, **Fernando,** for being patient and tender. Corinthians 13:4-7: "Love is patient, love is kind. It does not envy; it does not boast, it is not proud. It does not dishonor others; it is not self-seeking, it is not easily angered, it keeps no record of wrongs. Love does not delight in evil but rejoices with the truth. It always protects, always trusts, always hopes, always perseveres."